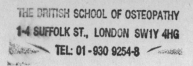

KATHARINA DALTON

Depression after childbirth

How to recognize and treat
postnatal illness

Oxford New York
OXFORD UNIVERSITY PRESS

Oxford University Press, Walton Street, Oxford OX2 6DP

Oxford New York Toronto
Delhi Bombay Calcutta Madras Karachi
Kuala Lumpur Singapore Hong Kong Tokyo
Nairobi Dar es Salaam Cape Town
Melbourne Auckland

and associated companies in
Beirut Berlin Ibadan Nicosia

Oxford is a trade mark of Oxford University Press

First published 1980 as an Oxford University Press
paperback and simultaneously in a hardback edition
Reprinted 1985

British Library Cataloguing in Publication Data

Dalton, Katharina Dorothea
Depression after childbirth.
1. Postnatal depression
I. Title
618.7 RG851 80–40664
ISBN 0-19-286008-9

Printed in Great Britain by
J. W. Arrowsmith Ltd, Bristol

Foreword

I am one of the thousands of women who have suffered from postnatal depression. I know, from my own experience, how unprepared you feel, and your family feels, when depression descends. I know how lonely I felt, surrounded by all the other happy, competent new mothers who clearly had not the slightest difficulty managing their homes, their work, their new babies, or themselves. So at least it looked to me at the time.

I also know from my own experience how humiliating it is to confess that one has had any kind of mental breakdown, no matter how temporary. Mental illness has become a taboo subject. When colleagues of mine decided to make a programme about postnatal depression, they could not find any woman in public life who was prepared to admit that she had suffered from it. But as a result of that programme, which was broadcast on BBC television, hundreds of letters poured in from women who were suffering from depression. The recurring theme in all those letters was that each woman had thought she was alone.

I took part in that programme, along with Mary Whitlock, who now runs the Meet-a-Mum Association of postnatal self-help support groups, and so did Dr Katharina Dalton. I am completely unqualified to judge her treatment of postnatal depression in medical terms. I am not, of course, a doctor. But I do know how tremendously impressive it was to meet her, because she has a complete understanding of depression, which feels like a physical illness and yet is so often dismissed as just another irrational female complaint.

Reading her book, I once again felt that enormous reassurance and relief. Here is someone who not only knows exactly what depression feels like, but has been able to treat it successfully. The silliest comment I ever heard about depression was that reading about it causes it. The reverse is true. Reading about postnatal depression in this book can only bring comfort to families who might otherwise feel isolated and hopeless. It makes those of us who have suffered from it feel less ashamed to admit it, and let us hope it makes those who dismiss it reconsider. After all, it is an illness that can and should be taken seriously. Thousands of women already have reason to thank Dr Dalton for her work. After this book many thousands more will have reason to thank her.

Esther Rantzen

Contents

Preface

This book is written for new mothers, fathers, grandparents, and all who unexpectedly come face to face with the problems of postnatal depression. It is hoped that this book will be considered essential reading for nurses, midwives, health visitors, and social workers so that they may understand the forces behind the many tears they see so unexpectedly in postnatal wards; that it will also be read by paramedical workers, sociologists; members of the self-help groups of MAMA and the National Childbirth Trust, Samaritans, and Depressives Anonymous to help them understand those who suffer in this way; and by probation officers, police, and magistrates so that sympathetic consideration may be given to those who unexpectedly and unintentionally behave in an irrational manner.

The subject matter stems from thirty years of listening, observing, patiently recording, and treating countless women, and recognizing the prolonged and unnecessary suffering which occurs in too many homes after the birth of a baby. It does not rely on long-held ideas, but on clinical observation, and presents a fresh viewpoint of an open mind. Charles Darwin spoke of the pleasures of observing and reasoning, and the results of such pleasures are echoed here.

An outline of medical treatment is given, but for my medical colleagues fuller details are to be found in *Premenstrual Syndrome and Progesterone Therapy* (2nd edition) published by William Heinemann Medical Books, London, 1984.

This work has only been made possible by the many women who have confided their deepest fears, hopes, anxieties, and feelings in utmost confidence. When using their quotations fictitious names have been given to ensure anonymity. My especial thanks go to Nancy for allowing me to use the unabridged version of her suffering in Chapter 7.

I would like once again to express my thanks to members of my family for teasing and bullying me to complete this work. To the Doctors Maureen and Michael Dalton for their comments and criticisms; to my daughter Mrs Wendy Holton for the hard work entailed in typing the manuscripts; to Mrs Anita Dalton for the artwork in the figures; and to Anthony Dalton Business Systems, Kenilworth, for the loan of equipment and photo-copying. I also wish to thank Mrs Elaine Jones, my hardworking secretary, for her typing of the numerous quotations. Acknow-ledgements for permission to publish figures which have already been published elsewhere go to Dr Yalom and his colleagues for Figure 1, and to Professor Kendall for Figure 10.

This work was completed in Holland, where with my husband, the Rev. Tom Dalton, I wrote and rewrote the chapters, which were so painstakingly ghosted and twisted round to intelligible English by my husband, ghostwriter. To him I owe my greatest thanks.

Katharina Dalton
7 July 1979

1
Introduction

A single baby's bootee with the cryptic message 'Get knitting' was posted from London to each set of future grandparents in Adelaide.

'Test positive – champagne at eight' was how one high-powered executive learned that he had been promoted to the ranks of a prospective grandfather.

These are two examples of how the good news of a confirmed pregnancy was announced. They were both young couples filled with excitement and happiness at the news of the confirmation of their fondest hope, a much-wanted baby. After the initial excitement at the realization that she is pregnant, the next few weeks are taken up with making decisions and planning for the future. The choice of a doctor, the place of birth, arrangements for housing, work commitment, and holiday schemes all call for consideration. Then come thoughts about the baby, wondering whether to bottle- or breast-feed, and further projections into the desirability of sending the child to play group or nursery school at an early age. But after the safe arrival, what then? No woman ever gives a thought to the chance of becoming the one in ten who is later affected by postnatal depression. This unexpected gloom, which can descend on a new mother and transform her whole personality, leads innumerable husbands to announce that 'She's never been the same since the birth of our baby'. Yet such a possibility is far from the thoughts of the happy young couples.

This is, of course, how it should be, for needless worrying about the one in ten chance throughout the pregnancy is obviously not a good thing. There are not many whose suffering is as severe and traumatic as some of the cases recounted here. Also, there is much that can be done about postnatal depression once it has been diagnosed. The earlier it is recognized the easier it is to treat, and that is one reason for writing this book, for there is far too great a silence about postnatal depression, which is considered to be merely the foibles of the weaker sex, just female fancies or feminine fantasies. It is an inexplicable problem which few people seem to understand, therefore it is considered wiser to sweep it under the carpet. It strikes without warning, bringing guilt, misery, and helplessness just when the young parents should be experiencing great happiness.

Postnatal depression is no respecter of persons. It attacks at random royalty, nobility, and famous personalities of screen and television, as well as the typist, the factory- and shop-worker, the flat-dweller, the squatter, and those caught in the poverty trap. The knowledge that Queen Victoria herself suffered is not much compensation. It strikes just the same at those who have a much-wanted child, including women who have endured years of attendance at the Infertility Clinics with relentless early morning temperature-taking, and those to whom the pregnancy was an unwelcome interruption of their well-ordered lives. It affects equally regular attenders at antenatal clinics and relaxation classes, and mothers who have spurned all medical help during their pregnancy. It comes unexpectedly into families who have a clean bill of health and have never before had to cope with a psychiatric illness, as well as the few who have a stillborn baby, and the many who have a healthy child. Unfortunately, postnatal depression can easily be missed and not recognized as an illness, but rather considered as a defect of personality which allows slovenliness, laziness, selfishness, and ingratitude to rise to the top.

Postnatal depression covers a range of afflictions, from sadness to suicide, which start after childbirth. They do not necessarily occur immediately, but within a few weeks or months, and they change the mother's behaviour, personality, and outlook. It is convenient to divide the afflictions into four groups; maternity blues, postnatal exhaustion, postnatal depression and puerperal psychosis. It is important to recognize that these four groups can merge imperceptibly into each other. Maternity blues are experienced by about half of all women after childbirth and result in unexpected episodes of profuse tears and mood swings. Postnatal exhaustion is a self-limiting tiredness, which may spoil the first few months of the baby's life. Postnatal depression occurs in one in ten women after childbirth and causes depression, exhaustion, irritability, and physical symptoms starting any time during the first year after the baby's birth. While in some mothers postnatal depression is self-limiting and is all forgotten about within weeks or months, in others the changed personality and life-style may persist for twenty or more years, and may gradually change into the premenstrual syndrome. When a woman is obviously mentally ill with such symptoms as delusions, hallucinations, threatening to take her own life or to injure the baby, and is in urgent need of hospital care for her own protection, then the illness is called 'puerperal psychosis', but fortunately such an illness is rare, only occurring in one in every 500 women. There is an excellent account of the working of the frenzied mind in this condition in 'Nancy's Tale', Chapter 7. Thus postnatal depression varies from the mildest of baby blues to the blackest of black depressions, although in press bulletins all forms tend to be lumped together under such euphemisms as 'nervous exhaustion', 'nervous debility', or merely as a 'breakdown'.

A recent BBC *Man Alive* television programme entitled 'Baby Blues to Breakdown' produced a deluge of letters from sufferers relating their personal experiences. They expressed relief that the subject had at last been opened up for discussion, and the hope that their husbands and relatives might appreciate their personal problems and have more understanding of their altered behaviour. Anna, who described herself as a long-suffering, overburdened housewife, pleaded:

'I am sure there are many of us needing help. I have suffered from these agonising, unrecognized, and untreated symptoms for what seems to be ages. It's so difficult to explain to others – no one really understands. It is a very bad thing and needs more understanding by everybody. Please educate everyone.'

Brenda, a social worker, asked:

'How many women are warned that they might suffer these miseries during the first few weeks of baby's arrival? How many of those who thrive during their pregnancy, and are filled with health and vivacity in spite of their awkward increasing shape, later think they are freaks when instead of sheer happiness at their perfect son they react with silent suffering and helpless depression?'

Other letters emphasized the seriousness of the problem:

'I tend to have difficult pregnancies and complicated labours, but that wouldn't deter me from having children. However with the depression experienced after this pregnancy I feel I could never have another one for this reason alone. I just long to get back to my own personality, my old energy and sex drive, and to be able to leave all this behind.'

Then there were the letters of those who had reached a point of desperation:

'I really need help. I can't spend the rest of my life as a psyche cripple. My problem is severe enough to prevent me living a normal life. I'm nearing the end of my rope.'

The majority of women suffering from postnatal depression do not even recognize that they are ill. They believe that they are just leading a lower quality of life bogged down by utter exhaustion and irritability – a sadly changed character. It is all too easy to blame their condition on to the extra work that the baby brings into their new life. However, once postnatal depression is recognized as a specific illness, different from typical depression, the outlook changes, for treatment needs to be specific and individually tailored – it is not enough to prescribe tranquillizers. Once the condition has been recognized and treated, the husband will be able to declare 'She's once more the woman I married.'

A doctor explained how, having had postnatal depression herself, her 'we and they' attitude to medicine had changed. Previously she had thought of 'we' as those with self-control, who don't let ourselves go, can control our temper and tears, and are eternally grateful for our healthy children. Afterwards she felt that women with postnatal depression were truly ill, not just ungrateful and lacking in moral fibre and self-control, and appreciated that they do not benefit from being told to 'pull yourself together'.

Unfortunately we cannot wait for all doctors to undergo that metamorphosis by personal suffering. The lack of understanding by the medical profession is understandable, for postnatal depression is an entity which falls between two specialities, obstetrics and psychiatry, but belongs to neither. It is seen and appreciated best in general practice. In *The Comprehensive Textbook of Psychiatry*, by A M Freedman and H Kaplan, a mere two pages out of a total of 1,620 are devoted to the subject. The budding obstetricians will regard *Integrated Obstetrics and Gynaecology for Postgraduates*, edited by Professor C J Dewhurst, as their Bible to see them through their higher qualifications, yet barely one page is devoted to the subject, although the editor does warn the reader that 'puerperal mental disorders is not an easy subject to grasp in all its intricacies'.

The obstetrician is responsible for the patient's care before delivery and during her short stay in hospital afterwards. But when a patient's behaviour appears odd or disturbed during the first postnatal days in the ward, it is often suggested that she should be discharged early in the hope that her home environment will enable her to recover quickly. If her behaviour then continues to deteriorate she will become the responsibility of the general practitioner, who may call in a psychiatrist if he feels it is necessary.

In the earlier and milder cases of postnatal depression the general practitioner will start treatment, and only when the treatment fails to bring an improvement or when the patient's condition deteriorates will the psychiatrist be called in. Therefore the psychiatrist will tend to see only those patients who deteriorate severely within a few days of the birth, and those whose illness has been protracted and who have had months or even years of treatment at the local surgery.

The general practitioner is, however, the only one who can watch and appreciate the gradual conversion of postnatal depression into the premenstrual syndrome, so he must always be aware of the possibility and listen to what the patient is trying to tell him. The responsibility, however, lies with the patient to bring clear evidence of the time-relationship of her symptoms to menstruation in the form of a carefully filled-in menstrual chart.

Many letters refer to the difficulty in approaching their doctor for help. Carol, a mother of two children in Yorkshire, wrote:

'I always get the same answer – that it is one of those things – it's something you have to live with – no one dies of it – and one doctor even suggested that it might be psychosomatic. Well after having realized what that meant, I was so upset and disgusted to think anyone could think you could imagine such an agonizing sickness. They just are not programmed to see a woman as a natural person.'

A husband, giving a full description of his wife's sufferings, ended:

'To make matters worse, although both her parents are doctors themselves, Diane has an apparent fear or phobia about visiting doctors or hospitals and has on certain occasions begged me not to "let anyone take her away"; it's almost as if she believed that she was no longer in normal control of herself.'

Continuous antenatal care is accepted as good medical practice, with regular monthly examinations in early pregnancy, increasing to weekly visits in the later months, thus ensuring a normal and safe delivery of a healthy baby. By comparison, postnatal care is perfunctory with little thought or attention being paid to the mental well-being of the mother, apart from a pat on the shoulder and an assurance that all will settle down soon. This is based on the assumption that all that matters is the delivery of a healthy baby, so once labour is completed all that is required is a postnatal examination at six weeks. Today it is appreciated that postnatal depression ranks as the commonest and most severe complication in the six months following the birth, so it is astonishing that no one has recognized the need for lengthy postnatal care, with at least one extra postnatal examination at three to six months. This should be psychologically orientated and aimed at diagnosing the 10 per cent of women with postnatal depression before the disability becomes chronic and too much damage is caused to the patient's life, her marriage, and her family. Postnatal depression is the principal complication of the puerperium, but will not necessarily be present at the time of the six weeks' examination.

The repercussions of the illness fall first upon the husband, who is already caring for the family and doing the housekeeping, and now has to take care of the new baby, often putting his own work and earning capacity in peril. Then they fall upon any other children in the family, and the new baby, who lose a happy home environment; while the personality change is all too often the last straw in breaking the relationship with the mother-in-law, who just fails to understand the predicament.

Even if doctors and the public are slow to recognize postnatal depression, it is recognized by the British law under the Infanticide Act of 1939 which states that a mother cannot be found guilty of the murder of her own child within twelve months of childbirth as 'the balance of her mind is disturbed by reason of her not having fully recovered from the effects of giving birth'. She can, however, be prosecuted for the lesser offence of manslaughter of her child, known as infanticide, for which she may be sentenced. Actually infanticide is quite rare – only nine women were convicted of the offence in 1983.

There may be historical reasons for the neglect of postnatal depression. For hundreds of years childbirth has been associated with a high death rate, especially due to puerperal pyrexia or septicaemia after childbirth. The open area in the womb to which the placenta was attached provides an inviting entry for infecting bacteria. There is little resistance to infection in the womb following delivery, so bacteria quickly reach the abdominal cavity, causing the dreaded peritonitis and death. One of the early warning signs of puerperal pyrexia is confusion, delusions, and hallucinations, with a rising temperature, and in the absence of effective treatment death was expected to follow within the next two days. It was Dr Ignas Semmelweiss (1818–56) who first stressed the importance of washing the hands after visiting the mortuary and before delivering the baby. That was in the days when medical students learned the art of delivering babies by practising in the mortuary on the bodies of women who had died in childbirth. His warning went unheeded in Budapest and later in Vienna, until Professor Joseph Lister at the Royal Infirmary, Glasgow, showed the vital importance of avoiding sepsis in surgical operations by the use of crude antiseptics such as carbolic acid. The death rate was further reduced dramatically by the discovery of penicillin by Professors Flemming and Florey, and since then by the discovery of many other antibiotics. Today puerperal pyrexia no longer spells death, although it is still a notifiable disease, which in England and Wales must be reported to the Department of Health and Social Security if the mother develops a temperature of 38°C (100·4°F) or over during the first fourteen days after the birth of her child. It has been the removal of puerperal pyrexia from the hazards of childbirth which has uncovered the problems of postnatal depression.

2
Maternity blues

Eileen was a telephone operator with an infectious laugh, guaranteed to keep the office happy, so not surprisingly, when she left for her maternity leave she was showered with gifts of baby-grows, baby powders, and lotions. She planned her nursery with care and was fully prepared for that greatest day of her life. The arrival of blue-eyed Adrian with his mop of black hair was witnessed by her husband Bill, a radio mechanic, who was normally squeamish at the sight of blood. This time it was different. They hugged, kissed, and congratulated each other on their big success, all 3 kilos (7 pounds) of him, during his first hour of life. The following evening the visiting hour was spent writing out the announcement cards, 'a bundle of Love has arrived', between more kisses and cuddles. But when Bill arrived on the third evening, clutching a bunch of red roses from their garden, Eileen had changed. Her face was no longer wreathed in smiles but instead tears washed away the carefully applied mascara. She cried at the sight of the flowers and, when that was over, there was another five minutes of crying as he proudly showed his letter of appointment to his new job. Then she grumbled about the food, the nurses, the other patients, the postman, and even the diminutive paper-boy who had come too early. Dutifully and lovingly Bill listened, encouraged, sympathized, and helped her over the day's trivialities. Within two days she was herself again, the brief episodes of tears had passed, and she was ready for discharge and for the start of a new life at home on the eighth day.

There is nothing unusual or different about that story. Eileen was like half the other women in her ward, suffering from maternity blues; the transient, self-limiting emotional upset which occurs during the days immediately following a birth. It may be known as 'baby', 'childbirth', 'puerperal', or 'postnatal' blues;

sometimes it is named as a reminder of the day of onset, such as the 'three', 'four', or 'five-day blues'; while others refer to it as the 'ten-day weepies', which represents how long this emotional upheaval usually lasts. In the nineteenth century it was known as 'milk fever' because it occurred during those days when milk was appearing in the breasts in quantity.

Crying is the most characteristic symptom of the blues; sobbing when she should be smiling joyously, or an unexpected flood of tears, perhaps lasting less than five minutes or continuing for hours on end. Sometimes she successfully controls the tears and is merely noticed to be sniffing. The crying is invariably accompanied by shame and later she is apologetic for having appeared in public with tears running down her cheeks. One wit of a husband suggested that the social services should be asked to provide professional shoulders for crying on! But in addition to tears there are more rapid mood changes from hearty laughter to uncontrolled sobbing.

A team of four psychiatrists from Stamford Medical School, led by Dr Irvin D Yalom, studied a group of thirty-nine women

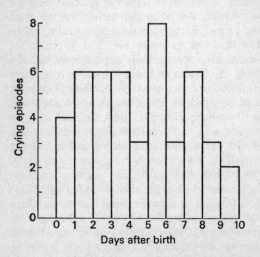

Fig. 1. Crying episodes in thirty-nine women after childbirth

both before delivery and for the first ten days after birth. They found that two-thirds had episodes of crying lasting at least five minutes during these ten days after the birth, while five women cried continuously for more than two hours. Figure 1 shows the days on which the episodes of crying occurred, with little difference during the first eight days and then a slight reduction. When this was compared with the ten-day period studied during pregnancy, their episodes of crying after the birth of the baby were three times higher than during pregnancy. Furthermore, during pregnancy the tears rarely lasted longer than five minutes.

The psychiatrists noticed that the women did not really cry from sadness, but for a variety of reasons, such as when they read the birth announcement; the ugliness of their baby; a sarcastic remark; when they received too much or too little attention from the nurses; when one of their room-mates left hospital; if they had insufficient milk; relief that the long-awaited labour was over; perhaps because they considered themselves a failure or had taken on more than they could cope with. Also they were always over-sensitive to minor rebuffs.

Frances, an ex-nurse from Surrey, who described herself as 'a thoroughly normal mother and housewife', wrote:

'The most depressing thing about puerperal blues is the way one is treated in hospital while suffering from the blues. I felt like a naughty child who'd misbehaved and must be chided or ignored till I behaved better, or worse still, was jollied/bullied along in the "get-up-and-forget-about-it" attitude. The treatment of new mothers in many hospitals leaves much to be desired anyway, though I do remember when I was nursing they were my least favourite patients as they weren't really ill.'

Young nurses are often embarrassed by the floods of tears from mothers who are older than they are. In a ward tears are infectious. In fact the postnatal ward is sometimes called the 'weeping ward', in contrast to the antenatal ward which is invariably a happy ward. The nurses in the postnatal ward know that if they happen to drop a cup or saucer the whole ward will be crying in unison within a few minutes of the crash. If one husband is so much as five minutes late at visiting time, all the mothers will react in sympathy.

Another difficulty for the new mother is that the nurses on the postnatal wards are not necessarily the same as the ones she had come to know so well on her frequent clinic visits. The bond that had been formed when the happy, carefree mother joked with the nurses during those months of antenatal examinations is abruptly broken when the new mother is admitted to the postnatal ward with her baby. Now in her emotional state she is called upon to establish new relationships with a fresh set of nurses and this can produce special problems for the mother.

Other symptoms of the blues, which may occur during these immediate postnatal days are fatigue, with poor concentration and slowness to learn, particularly such skills as bathing and feeding the baby, as well as confusion, anxiety (especially over the baby), and hostility directed towards the husband. One mother referred to it as 'a fit of the fed-ups which goes before it comes'. But these are all transient conditions, which have disappeared by the time of discharge from hospital or the time the midwife stops her home visits.

People who usually suffer from migraine are often freed from it during the last six months of pregnancy, but alas it often returns with a vengeance during the third to seventh day after childbirth.

The baby is sometimes a source of anxiety; the crying is disturbing to the new mother and there may be feeding difficulties which assume unreasonable proportions. The blotchy, red-faced newborn is very different from the filled-out, pink-cheeked baby of their dreams, and very different from the ones seen in photographs. The mother may be upset by the excessive interest and cooing over the baby when visitors come.

Dr Brice Pitt of the London Hospital realized that psychiatrists usually only see depressed women who are either acutely ill and admitted immediately after the birth, or chronically ill women several months later. He studied one hundred women, selected at random in the postnatal wards, and he interviewed them between the seventh and tenth day after their baby's birth. The blues were diagnosed if the women had felt tearful or depressed since the birth, and he noted that exactly half the women were suffering from the blues. In most of the women it was the usual fleeting, trivial disorder already referred to, but in six women the dejection lasted a month or more. Dr Pitt concluded:

'The presence of confusional features and the absence of personality predisposition or special psychological stresses, together suggest that the syndrome is organically determined. The lack of any significant association with infections or other ob-stetric complications leaves the most likely factor the profound endocrine change which follows parturition. The occurrence of two-thirds of the cases within four days of parturition, with a peak incidence on the third day, and the probably significant association with lactation problems among breast-feeders, suggest that the relevant change might be the precipitate fall in the progesterone and oestrogen levels post-partum.'

The possibility of a hormonal factor being responsible for postnatal depression is fully discussed in Chapter 12.

All who have seen the effects of postnatal depression emphasize the need for more information to be given to expectant mothers and fathers, and the need for sympathy by all those in contact with the new mother during the first few days after the birth. Treatment in the form of tranquillizers or antidepressants is certainly not called for, rather patience and understanding, for the predicament will soon vanish. The help that others can give, and guidance on the handling of those with the blues is contained in Chapter 14.

3
Endless exhaustion

A 46-year-old mother of two teenage sons was heard to declare:

'The traumatic effect of the black miseries and tiredness afterwards is worse than labour – the memory of them lasts much longer.'

When interviewing new patients and asking them about past pregnancies and whether there was any depression afterwards, you often find them hesitating and then awkwardly explaining that they felt awful for several months, exhausted because 'the birth took a lot out of me'. This postnatal exhaustion is really a mild form of depression. It may be self-limiting, lasting only three to six months, or it may be heralding a recognizable depression with irritability.

The mother feels exhausted and physically ill, with no energy or zest for living, and a desire to hide away and just sit without doing anything. She may excuse herself to her husband in the evening by saying that having a new baby is a full-time job, when in fact she crept back to bed after he went to work, didn't wash the breakfast things until four o'clock, and had sat in the lounge all afternoon lethargically watching television, yet hardly knowing what programme had been on. As one mother explained, 'I can't think, can't work, can't laugh, can't play and I just want to sit about all day.' Another mother recalled those days by saying:

'I can remember feeling so tired I was sure I was really ill, but my temperature was 35° or 36° C (95° or 96° F) – most disappointing.'

Tiredness covers both mental fatigue and physical exhaustion. It can be either healthy or unhealthy. There is that glowing, satisfying tiredness which follows a hard day's mental activity, the completion of a difficult essay or a stiff three-hour examination, and that same rewarding tiredness after a hard day's decorating, a strenuous round of golf, or jogging in the park. It is easily recognized when watching an athletics programme on television as we see the winner burst through the tape and then fall exhausted. Then there is the unhealthy tiredness which is not the result of hard work and is present in spite of a good night's sleep. It shows itself as mental apathy and a complete lack of physical energy.

This is the type of tiredness which characterizes postnatal exhaustion. The healthy tiredness is soon disposed of with relaxation, whereas all the sleep in the world won't ease the unhealthy variety.

Gail, a graduate laboratory worker until her pregnancy, described unhealthy tiredness by saying:

'I'm dead tired all day. There's no energy for unnecessary exertions like picking up a newspaper from the floor. Before I go into the kitchen I think of all the effort it will entail and almost count the steps there (I live in a small two-bedroomed flat). I have to push myself. None of my movements are natural and effortless like they used to be. I don't want anything to do or think about. I can't be bothered. Even to speak is an effort, it's easier to grunt a reply. It's like being in the half-awake, half-asleep state all day long.'

Lethargy is a dominant feature of this exhaustion, for all the mother's previous energy seems to have become transferred to the baby at the moment of birth, and is no longer within the mother to respond to the demands of everyday life.

A letter writer described it as 'a flatness which took a mighty long time to clear up', while a hairdresser, a mere six weeks after her child was born, apologized for her behaviour explaining:

'I've got everything I could wish for – a super husband, home, son, and daughter – both were planned and wanted; I desperately want to get well again – stop feeling so tired and enjoy it all again. The crux of it is that the energy has given up inside.'

That is true postnatal exhaustion. The exhaustion is both

mental and physical. A woman suffering from it will have problems in counting her change, doubling the ingredients in the recipe, sorting out times of trains or buses, and finding suitable dates for her holiday. If she's called upon to help with an older child's homework she will have the greatest difficulty in concentrating and working out any sums correctly. She will feel generally inadequate.

The pharmacists and health food stores rely on this postnatal exhaustion for their over-the-counter sales of iron and vitamin tablets and a selection of natural remedies guaranteed to cure exhaustion, but few of them ever are successful because postnatal exhaustion is due to a biochemical cause.

The recurring phrase heard from mothers with postnatal exhaustion is 'I can't cope'. This is echoed in Helen's letter:

'Even with ordinary things like cooking, changing a nappy, washing up, or preparing a meal, I just can't cope. They are tasks of enormous proportions. All this upsets me and makes me cry. My daughters used to have a clean dress to wear to school each day, now they just have to make do. I can't be bothered. I can't manage to do the cooking and the ironing as well, it has to wait for my husband at weekends, I just muddle through from day to day as best I can.'

This inability to cope is part of the illness and is not related to the woman's previous experience or abilities. The expression 'I just can't cope any more' is heard from those who are normally highly efficient and well organized as well as from those who are always in a muddle with their affairs. A sister in charge of a pre-mature baby unit in a busy provincial hospital worked for four years caring for the smallest of small babies, but found she couldn't cope when it came to her own healthy baby. It was also heard from a normally energetic, extraverted head of a nursery school, who had been controlling fifty children under 5 years of age and yet found it difficult to care for her only one.

One of Helen's worries was that her daughters had to rely on her husband doing the ironing, and she hated not having the energy to ensure that they were in clean dresses each day for school. But the mother herself also ceases to be bothered about her own appearance and although she is aware that her standards have deteriorated she is quite unable to do anything about it.

A mother with a healthy son of 4 months wrote:

'My appearance has gone to pot because I can't seem to be bothered, although I know how much my husband would like to see the old me. Even my tremendous love for my husband does not seem to prod me into action.'

Sleep is a recurring problem for women with postnatal exhaustion. The patients have an endless yearning for sleep and can never get enough. They can sleep all day and all night. Even when a kind husband, relation, or friend offers to be responsible for looking after the baby at night, and they have a full twelve hours undisturbed sleep, they will still be yearning for more. In this way postnatal depression differs from the typical depressive illness where the patient goes to sleep but then wakes early at 3, 4, or 5 am, and lies awake depressed and anxious until it's time to get up.

When mothers are recalling the days of exhaustion after the birth, it is frequently prefaced by the remark: 'But then mine was a crying baby – he never stopped crying day or night.' There can be little doubt that a ceaselessly crying baby is exhausting. When you have done all the things that the baby books tell you to do to stop the baby crying, and he still persists, it can be most frustrating. But a crying baby may be reacting to the exhausted mother. It is the old chicken-and-egg situation, which comes first? How often have you handed the baby's care over to someone else for a few hours, or perhaps overnight, and that person hands him back with the innocent comment 'I haven't heard a squeak from him the whole time'? Was the baby reacting to firmness, confidence, and infinite patience?

The social workers, health visitors, and district nurses are taught to keep an eye open for mothers showing the early signs of postnatal depression, and usually it isn't a very difficult exercise. A mother is suspect if she misses her postnatal appointment or the clinic appointment for her child's jabs; she's confused and can't organize herself to get to the clinic on time. A home visit reveals the patient as quite different from the carefully made-up, well-coiffured lady who attended the antenatal clinic. She's now dishevelled with no make-up, and no recent signs of a shampoo and set. The home is a bit of a muddle with the baby's clothes on the floor, a pile of nappies waiting to be washed, and several used cups on the draining board. The visitor will be offered a cup of tea or coffee, and the young mother will happily sit down and drink her fourth mug that morning. She will complain of her need for sleep, even though her head hit the pillow at seven the night before and she didn't stir until her husband brought the tea at nine that morning. She needs help, and it is the health visitor's task to organize medical treatment, plus a home help until she is able to cope herself.

The excessive exhaustion may result from the body's supply of potassium being too low. This can result from a poor diet, from the kidney removing too much potassium and passing it out in the urine, or from the use of diuretic tablets (to encourage the flow of urine). It can easily be recognized by a simple blood test, and remedied by increasing the consumption of potassium-rich foods, especially bananas and tomato- or orange-juice, or by taking potassium tablets.

Sometimes the exhaustion may be due to causes other than depression, such as thyroid deficiency. During pregnancy the pituitary gland is responsible for the secretion of prolactin which prepares the breasts for lactation, and after labour for breast-feeding. But this is not the only hormone with which the pituitary gland is concerned; it is also responsible for the thyroid, adrenals, and pancreas. Sometimes, following the sudden switch-round of hormones at labour, there is not enough of the chemical messenger called the 'thyroid stimulating hormone'. This is the hormone which passes from the pituitary gland, situated at the base of the brain to the thyroid gland, situated at the front of the neck: it tells the thyroid gland to produce its special hormones such as thyroxine. These thyroid hormones are used to control the speed at which the body works. If there is insufficient thyroid hormone the body works slowly and the mother falls asleep at any time of the day or night; she feels cold, with dry skin and lank hair which tends to fall out, and has a slow pulse. A simple blood test will quickly measure the level of thyroid stimulating hormone, and also test the functioning of the thyroid gland to help the doctor decide whether the gland is working normally. If there is a deficiency, the treatment will also be simple and merely consists of taking one to three tablets daily of a thyroid hormone, such as thyroxine.

Another possible reason for a mother feeling exhausted after childbirth is anaemia. There may have been a haemorrhage at the time of delivery, and if there was not enough iron in her body's stores to replenish the blood loss, there may be anaemia. This can be diagnosed by another cheap and easy blood test, and if any anaemia exists this can be corrected by giving iron.

Usually the exhaustion, which is a mild form of depression, is self-limiting and is eased before the first six months are over, but occasionally it gets worse and other features of postnatal depression develop, especially irritability. A young shop worker recalled the first few weeks after her twins were born:

'I was so flaked-out and tired I couldn't rise to anger then – I was far too tired and sleepy, but after a few months I was throwing things and hitting the kids.'

4
Postnatal depression

Depression is an illness which occurs in men, women, and children, and at all ages. It is characterized by gloom, despondency, and despair. Depression has been described as a 'disease of loss', and indeed it really is so, for there is a loss of happiness, pleasure, interests, and enthusiasm, as well as loss of ability to concentrate, to remember, and to think clearly, also the loss of bodily functions like sleep, appetite, weight control, and bowel movement (Figure 2). Sometimes depression is divided into two types of illness; it is called 'reactive' if it is the result of an obvious cause of sadness, such as after a bereavement, redundancy, or divorce, and 'endogenous' when it occurs for no apparent reason. But this differentiation is not really very important as both types need the same methods of treatment.

Depression can also be an emotion or sadness. It is a normal physiological emotion which all healthy normal people experience in the course of their lives. If we learn that one of our friends has been killed in a road accident, or their house has been burnt down, we would naturally feel depressed, sad, and unhappy, but we would not necessarily be ill or suffer from the loss of any abilities or bodily functions as shown in Figure 2, nor would we need treatment.

The medical fraternity appreciate the confusion caused by the word 'depression', and sometimes they prefer to talk about a 'depressive illness' instead. Until the early part of this century doctors used the word 'melancholia' to describe a depressive illness.

Postnatal depression has some characteristics which are different from those usually found in typical depression, and so it is known as 'atypical' (meaning not typical). This is an important distinction, as we shall see later, because the commonly pre-

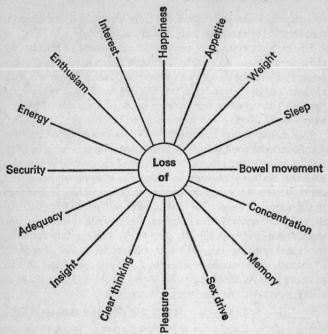

Fig. 2. Depression is a disease of loss

scribed antidepressant drugs are effective for typical depression, but special types of drugs are more effective for atypical depression.

Depression can start at any age in life, but postnatal depression is atypical because it can only start after a pregnancy. Irritability is a marked feature of postnatal depression, but not necessarily present in typical depression. Because irritability is such an important symptom in postnatal depression it is dealt with separately in Chapter 5.

In typical depression the patient has difficulty with sleeping. He or she may get off to sleep but then characteristically has early morning waking and lies awake in utter despair until it's time to get up. On the contrary, women with postnatal depression have a yearning for sleep and never get enough. They sleep heavily, even though they wake instantly if the baby wakes, and can sleep on throughout the morning, and indeed the whole day.

The early mornings are usually the worst time of the day for those with typical depression, and then they improve as the day goes on. By contrast, women with postnatal depression are often at their best in the morning, but the depression and inability to cope with the routine work comes on during the day. They feel worse in the evening and want to go to bed early.

Typical depression is characterized by a loss of appetite with a revulsion from food, which in turn leads to loss of weight, often 5 to 15 kilos (1 or 2 stones) in a matter of months. This is such a common finding that when the doctor is treating someone with depression he will gauge the success or failure of his treatment by the amount of weight the patient has gained. With postnatal depression the problem is different, the appetite is increased and the woman is always thirsty, continually tucking into fattening foods and drinking mugs of tea or coffee to while away her hours of solitude. She may have odd cravings when she gorges on bars of chocolate, stacks of toast and honey, or piles of doughnuts or sticky buns. A Canadian mother described:

'. . . the solicitude of my friends and relations over my quaint eating habits. There is complete disinterest in foods at certain times but binges inevitably follow. I wake up at night hungry and grab whatever is in sight. I hide fudge about the house so that I know where to find it when it's needed. I can't help gorging it even when I'm ready to bust.'

The result of the increased appetite is that sufferers rapidly gain weight, even within a month or two they are heavier than they were when their final weight was taken at the clinic a day or two before the baby was born. It is known as 'maternal obesity' with the fat centred especially around the abdomen, but with thin wrists and ankles. Some women refer to their increasing girth as 'bloatedness' or 'water retention' but this is not fluid retention, it is true fat or adiposity. One woman described how 'nowadays I feel like an old waterlogged hag – like death warmed up'. Failure to appreciate that this abnormal appetite and weight gain is part of postnatal depression may be another cause of marital disharmony, for there is always the thoughtless husband who declares bluntly: 'I don't like obese women'.

One physical sign which is not always present, but which, if seen, is positively diagnostic of postnatal depression, is the presence of milk in the breast two or more months after breast-feeding has stopped. This never occurs in typical depression. Such milk in the breast is called 'galactorrhoea' or 'inappropriate lactation'. One mother of a 4-year-old daughter asked: 'What about the milk which is still oozing out of my breasts?'

Galactorrhoea occurs when there is too much of one of the pituitary hormones called prolactin. One of the many functions of prolactin is to prepare the breasts for lactation during pregnancy, and later to stimulate the breast milk when breast-feeding occurs. So in pregnancy and during breast-feeding there is a high level of prolactin in the blood, but this should diminish when breast-feeding stops and return to the level of a non-pregnant woman. A blood test can recognize women with a high level of prolactin in their blood, even though they are not breast-feeding. Treatment is with the drug bromocriptine, but more about that on page 120.

By now it is hoped that the reader will appreciate that postnatal depression is not the same as typical depression, but a special type which needs special treatment.

There is the inevitable confusion with the word 'depression' for this suggests that it's all in the mind, whereas to the sufferer it's all in the body. They feel physically ill, and are indeed ill, they are sure that theirs must be a real illness, which will readily show up on blood tests or X-rays. It is an illness due to a biochemical abnormality in the brain, which controls the workings of the body, and also a biochemical abnormality in the blood which perfuses all the tissues of the body. In postnatal depression it is usual to hear such expressions as:

'I ache all over.'

'There's a continual aching of my muscles and bones.'

'I'm tender all over, especially in my breasts. I bruise easily and feel generally out of sorts.'

This is how one young mother described her experiences:

'When I am depressed I can't sleep enough at night, so I feel I could sleep all day. Really exhausted, very weepy and can't stop crying, can't think straight, nothing goes right, and I'm really terribly irritable and short-tempered. I feel I never will get better, everything is in a hopeless mess. I feel very sick and sometimes retch and feel queasy. Don't want to have anything to do or think about, just no energy for this. I get very hot spells at times and feel faint. I hurt everywhere and cannot cope, but all the tests and examinations by my good old family Doc, I am told, are quite alright. So I must be normal.'

Dizziness, or vertigo, is another common symptom which makes mothers think they are really physically ill, as suggested by this extract from Janet's letter:

'Suddenly the swimming starts with the entire room going round. I somehow lose my equilibrium. I have to hold my head and keep quite still. I never mention this to anyone as I'm terrified I have a brain tumour or something else horrible.'

Doctors recognize that women rarely come along to the surgery saying they're depressed, but by careful questioning they can get round to the problem. They may ask 'Are you as happy as you used to be?', or more vaguely 'How's life – are you enjoying things?' These are good opportunities for the young mother to open up and discuss her problems, how the black cloud hangs over her life, how everything is getting on top of her, or the difficulty in coping with the new baby, as well as the housework, shopping, and husband. Or they may ask if they are lonely, allowing the young mothers to talk about the difficulties of socializing, getting on with others, getting confused, and saying the wrong thing. Or sometimes the more pointed question is asked: 'Have you changed since having baby?'

Women in certain cultures regard the use of the word 'depression', in regard to themselves, as an insult. It is rather like asking someone if they are a slut, or lazy, or dirty, so the word is best avoided. If necessary it is better to speak of a depressive illness or melancholia.

All too often the mother feels vaguely ill and different, but doesn't quite know what has happened or how to seek help.

29-year-old Kathleen was in this predicament, and told me how she had been to the doctor's surgery on four occasions to ask for help, but somehow had failed. First she asked about the scaling on her baby's scalp, accepted a prescription and left the surgery before realizing she hadn't got down to the real problem. A week or two later she went to the health centre and mentioned her cough. Her chest was examined and she was assured that all was well. She tried a more direct approach on her next visit, and spoke about her tiredness and desire to sleep all day. She was given the necessary form to take to the local hospital for a blood test. The following week she was told her blood test was 100 per cent, wasn't she lucky? She wasn't anaemic and wouldn't need to take any more iron tablets. It was nearly a month later, with her son Charles now 9 months, that she burst into tears and flew off the handle because the receptionist had muddled up her appointment. Thus finally by her tears she got her message over to the doctor. Kathleen was roused to anger and could explain how her whole life had changed; she had lost her *joie de vivre*, felt inadequate, hopeless, and couldn't make decisions. She confessed: 'I'm a Christian woman and am ashamed of my behaviour. I can't understand what's happening to me.' There had indeed been a change in Kathleen, who'd been a personal assistant to a company director, one of the jet set, and it had been her task to organize and co-ordinate arrangements for his international tours. The tours, hotels, tickets, and flights had always been planned flawlessly.

Under the heading 'I suffered too', the popular television personality, Esther Rantzen, described in the magazine *Woman* her attack of afterbaby blues:

'Yes, I'm lucky. A great job, a loving husband, a nanny to look after the baby . . . but I was utterly defenceless when it happened to me. For a month it was utter hell. I felt as if I was going insane. I have heard myself shouting at my husband in an unforgivable way and yelling that I must see a doctor, that I was going mad. There were awful attacks of shaking, stumbling, and trembling.

I suffered from what I call "mind slip". I couldn't concentrate. I could not even dictate letters because I was getting my words mixed up. It was as if I'd lost a part of myself.

I was one of the lucky ones, though. I managed to get out of it by talking over my feelings with everyone from my husband, friends, and family, to my health visitor who was wonderful, and a marvellous doctor came round and listened. But all the same I felt guilty about taking up so much professional time.'

Dr Stuart Carne, a London general practitioner, spoke at the Royal Society of Medicine about the recognition of depression in a mother who brought in a baby with persistent vomiting for which no cause could be found. By the treatment of the mother's depression the baby's vomiting was stopped.

Women are all different. Different genetically, with different childhood environments and experiences, different social classes and intelligencies, and they all look different. It is therefore not surprising that the way they are affected by this 'disease of loss' will vary, some putting greater stress on some losses than others. The very descriptions they give of their lowered moods vary, including such statements as:

'A feeling of being detached from everyone and everything around me. It's like living in a bubble. I'm near to things yet far away.'

'It's a cosmic melancholy.'

'I can't relieve the feeling of sadness. Every item in the news-paper seems to be a sob story and starts me off weeping.'

The letter from Linda described how for her it was indeed a disease of loss, as she wrote:

'I have had so many bouts of deep depression. I have been in hospital twice because I swallowed an overdose of tablets, the last occasion in September of last year. Does anyone really know what it is like to feel suicidal, to have cups falling out of your hand, to feel too lazy to pick things up, to sit and just watch things happen that you can do nothing about.'

Mary was also at the end of her tether when she wrote:

'Everything is closing in on me. No one understands. Mine are tears of anger. I break down in floods of tears in the streets, shops, and other inconvenient places. I feel I have tried everything and am afraid I shall get to the point where I will give up trying and succumb to my violent tendencies, either towards myself or someone else.'

Nina, whose baby is now 8 months, showed a mixture of depression and irritability when she wrote:

'Suddenly I feel heavy depressions, I'm irritated with my husband and children. I start looking for quarrels; several times I feel hopeless, start weeping on my own, gasping for breath and wish myself dead. Then I'm afraid to be alive, I desire to be dead and start to think how it is possible to die (often I have suicide feelings). Often I have headaches and pain in the back, particularly when I'm reading, thinking, or studying. During the depressions I dislike women and I'm irritated by little things. When these feelings go on for a day and sometimes more days I'm afraid to meet other people, eg the people in my husband's office. Afterwards I myself do not understand my own behaviour.'

Suicide is an ever-present possibility. It is a continual fear to the sufferer, and all those who are close to someone who is in the throes of a depressive illness should keep the danger in the forefront of their minds. It is all too easy to pick up and swallow some readily available tablets. Most attempts are cries for help and can succeed in focusing attention upon the real dilemma of the new mother, which then leads to positive treatment, adequate help, and a new life. On other occasions the real problem is not considered, it is seen as a foolish attempt by a stupid woman, a superficial view is taken of the incident and a recurrence of the attempt is inevitable. Sometimes the end result is worse than the depression, as one mother found out: 'Last year after a stupid suicide effort I ended up with three months in plaster because of a broken leg.'

The depression brings with it a desire to withdraw from one's surroundings, to become detached, avoid socializing and making contact with other people. Doctors are used to hearing phrases like 'all I want to do is run away and hide myself in a corner'.

An accountant living in Cornwall wrote:

'I have managed not to let it interfere with my life too much, although it has affected my social life. I used to be the secretary of the local bridge club and the Women's Institute and was responsible for arranging the meetings. Now I avoid mixing socially and I know this has made me very difficult to live with. Everybody thinks it's because of the babysitting problem, but really it is that I don't want to see anyone anymore.'

The loss of confidence which occurs in depression is noticed by those who were previously leaders in their spheres and were extroverts. Olive, a science teacher, explained:

'I have completely lost all confidence in looking after my baby, and of course could not breast-feed her, which really upset me. I don't seem to cook so well and am frightened of trying out any new recipes. I dare not attempt dressmaking any more for fear that I will spoil the material by cutting it out wrongly, yet I have been dressmaking for the last ten years.'

The mental confusion poses a problem and makes women frightened of going out, afraid that they will hand out the wrong fares on the buses, or absent-mindedly walk out of a shop without paying. In an effort to avoid others noticing their confusion they'll rush into a shop, pick up the nearest article, pay for it, and hurry out. Only later do they realize that it's the wrong size, they've bought too little or too much, or that it's suitable only for cats or dogs, and not for babies.

A Nigerian mother of two children was found guilty of shoplifting only ten days after having a Caesarean operation to deliver her baby. It seems she picked up three baby's dresses, but only paid for two. One cannot help wondering why a mother was allowed out shopping alone so soon after a major operation. More important one asks: 'Was there a woman magistrate on the bench, and had she ever had children?'

It is not surprising that many new mothers end up by being frightened of themselves and of their own actions, for they cannot understand what is going on within them. They are frightened of taking their own lives, frightened of going out shopping, frightened of hurting the baby, or dropping him, of drowning him in the bath, and even frightened of his crying. In the end they are frightened of their own company, and of being alone. They will not let their husbands out of their sight. The young mother will cry when her husband attempts to go to work in the morning, and if he succeeds she will phone him and call him home from work. After a while it is only the most patient of employers who can put up with the husband's continual absences. Penny, a mother in this type of predicament, pleaded:

'I don't know what will happen if someone doesn't help me soon. I'm seriously afraid I will lose my husband, he will lose his job. I will wreck the car and damage the children's lives for ever. I am not fit to live with.'

Rejection of the baby and hostility towards him, is another problem which may arise in postnatal depression. Often one hears remarks, uttered in strictest confidence, which explain this predicament. A distraught mother might use such phrases as:

'I don't love him any more.'

'I'm emotionally flat about him – he doesn't move me.'

'I can't understand it – I looked forward so much to his arrival and now I can't stand him. I even attended doctors for five years to have him.'

'He's repulsive.'

'I wish he'd go away – I don't want my baby.'

A Jewess, who had three daughters without any problems afterwards then gave birth to her first son which was followed by an unpleasant depression, explained: 'My greatest wish was to give my husband a son. I've done that now, but I hate him and am even frightened of him.'

It used to be thought that inability to love a baby could lead to depression, but the opposite is true. It is the very depression which blunts the love for the much-wanted baby.

When the pregnancy has been happily anticipated and then the rejection and loss of love for the baby occurs it is always a sign that the mother is ill and in need of medical help, for doctors can help to correct the situation and assist the mother's natural love to return. The feelings of rejection also give rise to unpleasant feelings of guilt, so that it becomes a deep secret, and may be hidden from those nearest and dearest to her. It calls for careful consideration and sympathetic handling by the husband and other members of the family.

At a medical meeting dealing with marriage guidance the speaker stated that of all the medical causes of marital breakdown postnatal depression topped the list. He was not just referring to recent postnatal depression, but the illness which went on for twenty years going on to become the premenstrual syndrome. He asked 'How often does the first interview contain the husband's statement "She's never been the same since the baby was born?"' The audience was advised that when there was a possibility that the marital disharmony stemmed from the birth of a child, it was an indication for a full medical interview with the mother to exclude the possibility of postnatal depression or the premenstrual syndrome. He stated that if either postnatal depression or the premenstrual syndrome were present, specific treatment was more likely to heal the rift in the marriage than further interviews with counsellors.

Of course it is always possible for women, particularly those who have had a previous typical depressive illness when not pregnant, to have a recurrence of their typical depression during the first year after childbirth. They will then have the characteristic features of typical depression rather than those of postnatal depression. It is for the doctor to differentiate the two types, for the choice of treatment will depend on the type of depression.

5
Postnatal irritability

Everyone suffers from irritability at some time in his or her life, for it is a natural outlet for frustration, and any violence that may be involved is directed towards the cause of the irritation. In this chapter, however, we are dealing with an irritation which, when it breaks out into violence, is quite indiscriminate in its object of attack. It is, above all, an irritability which is quite out of keeping with the person's character and all too often ends in violence, both verbal and physical, followed by tears.

A distraught mother described the change in her daughter, Susan, who had previously been the head of the Art Department at a school:

'The destructive urge is not limited to self-destruction but includes others, such as the husband and children, and also material things like throwing the iron, the saucepans, or even the sewing machine across the room. It also includes attempts at arson – setting alight her own home, her favourite books, and her love-letters.'

It has already been stated that irritability is an important symptom of postnatal depression. This importance is derived from its diagnostic value, for the irritability described above is quite different from that associated with typical depression and therefore responds to a quite different treatment. It also has another quite important aspect, which is its similarity in every way to the irritability of the premenstrual syndrome. This syndrome has one characteristic feature, the triple symptoms of tiredness, irritability, and depression which together make up the 'tension' of premenstrual tension, the commonest symptom of the premenstrual syndrome. The premenstrual syndrome and tension are of hormonal origin and are successfully treated with the responsible hormone.

It is no coincidence that the premenstrual syndrome often evolves out of postnatal depression, as you will learn in Chapter 11, for postnatal depression has the same three symptoms. Calmness can be restored by treatment with progesterone (Chapter 15).

The irritability does not necessarily start immediately after birth, but develops slowly over the next few months, gradually masking the importance of exhaustion and depression. The irritability itself is variable in its intensity in each individual and may show itself as a complete and thoroughly destructive outburst, but whatever the intensity it is not within the patient's power to completely control it. Valerie, a 20-year-old mother, wrote:

'I am as ratty and quarrelsome as ever, ranging from petty squabbles to occasional violent outbursts which affect our home for days. I really do feel guilty about this but it never helps to control my temper. Nothing gets done in the house and my bookwork suffers and I can't concentrate and I get confused. I hide myself away in shame, convinced that every other woman in the world is coping splendidly.'

A more violent outbreak is described by Tina, whose twins are now 14 months old. She realized:

'For quite a while now I have been behaving outrageously. I decided to go to the University Health Centre and get psychiatric help, for after a specially bad crisis I thought I was mad. I had been breaking the bathroom scales by jumping on it with an incredible rage, then I had taken ten sleeping tablets to quieten me down and slept for sixty hours, and all because the dog had eaten half of my coat.'

The irritability also shows itself in emotional swings from anger to distress, which of course can be seen in Tina's case, for after smashing the bathroom scales she took ten sleeping tablets to quieten herself, and finished up with a two-and-a-half days' sleep. The aggressive outbursts are always a potential danger to people outside the family circle, although the mother seems to try hard to keep it within the home. This, in itself, puts an enormous strain on the husband, as this account reveals in which a husband describes his wife's emotional swings:

'She is apparently unable to control her reactions and attitudes when we are together, although to the best of my knowledge she has never displayed such extreme symptoms in the presence of other people. However, there are now almost regular and pre-dictable times when we are alone that she will break down com-pletely – displaying the extremes of anger and distress in a most alarming manner. During the past week, she has had four such major outbursts which have involved shouting and screaming, attempted physical violence towards me and very long periods of apparently hysterical and uncontrollable sobbing. Indeed I do not think that this word correctly describes her action as it seems to me not to be crying in the conventional sense of the word. She moves her arms and legs in a regular rhythmic motion and gasps and gulps uncontrollably. This often happens in the evening or at night, though daytime scenes have also occurred when we work together; usually one of these outbursts lasts for between half-an-hour to an hour-and-a-half, always starting with initial anger, leading to violence, and thereafter the inevitable breakdown into tears and sobbing.'

Frequently these attacks of irritability end up with uncontroll-able sobbing which seems to resolve the irritability for a while. The quarrelsome aspect is always of constant concern for those women who, before pregnancy, held down posts calling for ad-ministrative and executive ability. The sudden change in temper is alarming to them, whereas previously they were slow to anger, now they find they flare up at the slightest provocation. They find the simple remedies for self-control no longer work. Here are two examples from civil servants:

'I'm hostile to the world, acting like Dracula, and completely out of control. The least thing upsets me and I don't want to make decisions (not always possible to defer). At times I could literally grind my teeth, but to no purpose.'

'I'm impatient with my elderly father and occasionally break china and glass, although I loathe violence and aggression. I am dissatisfied with my life-style and environment. I find it is impossible to overcome this by the conscious effort of trying to count my blessings.'

This is because the irritability is of chemical origin, and the mother soon finds it is not so easy to control by psychological methods, such as grinding her teeth, counting her blessings, or trying to look upon the bright side. One mother used to count up to ten before giving her 6- and 4-year-old daughters a well-deserved smack. In no time they'd learnt the difference between 'nine' and 'ten' and would continue misbehaving until mother reached 'nine'. So mother started counting up to ten in French, then German, and then Dutch. The children had their first foreign language lessons, but I doubt if it really helped mother.

The outburst is limited to the immediate present with complete blindness as to its future effect, as reflected in the accounts of two women. One said: 'I'd been crying, I smashed up the kitchen. I screamed in fury and then was shattered.'

The other said: 'Pity the poor dog. I always kick him first.'

The one gave no thought to the mess that would have to be cleared up, nor was the other concerned as to whether the dog would bark less in future.

The irritability is reflected on the husband, for too often he is at the wrong end of his wife's bad temper. He finds she has changed from the elated, vivacious person she was during pregnancy into the ever-moaning bitch of today. Can you blame him if he stops in for a quick pick-me-up on his journey home before he faces another irrational flow of verbal abuse or physical danger? All too often the wife knows what's happening but can do little about it. Alison wrote:

'Don is not a terrible ogre – he is a decent man and he loves me. He was a salesman for a pharmaceutical firm and understands quite a lot of medical things, but he does not understand why sometimes I pick fights and make him the butt of my bad humour.'

These emotional swings, the quarrelsomeness, violence, and lack of tolerance, build up a constant sense of fear in the postnatally depressed mother who, recognizing her inability to control these waves of changing emotions, becomes frightened of herself. One concerned mother wrote about her daughter:

'Barbara is, I think, slightly better but still suffers bad fits of depression and of course it is not the best situation to be alone with a small child all day and every day – she is an intelligent person and needs some stimulation and conversation. She does love Frank very much – he is also bright and intelligent – but I know she is frightened of herself at times, of these sudden bouts of tempers and going out of control, and shouting etc, or striking the child.'

In one couple the husband was infertile. He was found on examination to have no sperms, so the wife had artificial insemination. In due course the baby arrived, but then the mother developed postnatal depression with irritability so bad that in her own words: 'I could have battered him each time he would not stop crying.'

Sometimes postnatal depression does not start until a later pregnancy, so that the older children are already well adjusted to a happy family life, and then the mother's character changes. Getting children to appreciate the problems that the illness brings is indeed difficult and not always successful.

Christine wrote:

'I have two older children and they are suffering from my lack of tolerance and general snappiness. Consequently, my eldest child, Graham, who has a problem of his own, has become introverted and withdrawn. It must be dreadful not to have a cheerful Mummy. And yet I try so hard, but cannot succeed.'

Another wrote in the same vein, ending:

'I now realize that if the downs continue it will not only affect a happy marriage, but it will in all likelihood damage my own daughter's security as well.'

So by now you are well aware of the effect of irritability and why it is considered such an important symptom, but what can be done about it? This question is dealt with in Chapter 15, although Chapter 14 deals with ways in which others can help.

Consideration needs to be given to the factors that act as a stimulus to postnatal irritability. Noise can be an irritant, especially high-pitched sounds, but the noise itself seems less important than its possible source, consequently the cries of the baby are often claimed to be the stimulus that sets off the irritability. Certainly the never-ending crying of the baby with which the mother cannot cope produces a potentially dangerous situation. When the mother is overcome by a sudden aggressive outburst the urge to hurt the helpless weakling may be extremely difficult to suppress. Tales of baby-battering so shock the public that young mothers dare not confide their fears that they might one day injure their own child. In practice one finds that the truth of whether a mother has ever hurt her child takes some time to reveal, it does not necessarily emerge at the first few interviews. Indeed it was only after Debby had been under my care for twelve months, for the treatment of postnatal depression which had merged into the premenstrual syndrome, that she thanked me for the greatest benefit the treatment had brought. She said she had not hit even one of her four children once during the last year. At last she confessed that her children had many unnecessary bruises on their limbs, which had been inflicted by her, and she had even put her hands around her 16-month-old son to strangle him, but somehow she had avoided it at the last minute. Her greatest fear was that the children she loved so much might be taken into care.

The last straw, and the factor which finally releases the explosive outburst, is often the drop in blood sugar. As is explained on page 112, after birth and later on, before menstruation, there may be an alteration in the ability of the body to cope with changes in the varying amount of sugar in the blood. If there has been too long an interval without food (or more particularly without either sugar or starchy foods) then the body reacts and corrects the blood sugar level by spurting out adrenalin to release some extra sugar from the body's stores and raise the blood sugar level again. As every schoolchild learns in biology, adrenalin is the hormone of 'fight, fright, and flight', so when the adrenalin is suddenly poured into a woman's blood it may cause her to fight in fury. A mother who is liable to bouts of irritability would be advised to abandon her rigid old-fashioned Victorian ideals of 'no food between meals', and 'only three meals a day' in favour of a 'little and often' regime to restore happiness in the home.

If the irritability, quarrels, and aggressive behaviour are not recognized as an illness they can cause permanent damage to relationships and make lifelong enemies. Perhaps it is the much maligned mother-in-law who has the greatest difficulty in appreciating the true situation. If she sees her own son suffer from an apparently jealous and spoilt wife who expects him to do all the fetching and carrying, and who doesn't visit his parents, can she really be blamed for speaking her mind and telling her daughter-in-law how lazy and ungrateful she is? Greater understanding of the whole problem of postnatal depression is the real answer.

When the irritability is recognized as part of postnatal depression it can be treated specifically with gratifying results. However, if it is seen in isolation there is a natural temptation to treat it with sedatives or tranquillizers, indeed it is often the patient who asks for sedation. Unfortunately depression and exhaustion are already present and nothing is achieved by giving more sedatives to a woman who is already oversedated by her illness. One has sympathy with Elaine who wrote:

'When I take enough sedatives or tranquillizers to calm me down I walk around in a fog like some kind of zombie. I can't get my housework done, much less drive a car. I keep telling the doctor he's treating the symptoms and not the cause. And he just pats my head and smiles. It's maddening.'

6
Puerperal psychosis

The most severe form of baby blues occurs in the form of puerperal psychosis. This is a mental illness with a 'frenzied mind', in which the patient has lost contact with reality. She may be confused, deluded, irrational, or hallucinatory. It is the type of illness where even the husband and family appreciate that the mother is ill and badly in need of medical treatment. Fortunately it is a rare complication with only one mother in 200 to 500 births succumbing to the condition. The psychiatrists divide the psychotic illnesses into organic, schizophrenic, depressive, and manic, and in the past there was also the toxic delirium which included puerperal pyrexia but today it is rare, as deadly infections no longer occur in our sterile delivery rooms, and if they do we have effective antibiotics with which to control them. These psychotic illnesses may occur in men and women, and do not only happen after childbirth.

Hospitalization is essential for all but a very few women. It is needed for the patient's sake so that she may recover as speedily as possible, for her own safety, and to protect the lives of others, especially the baby.

Two days after the birth of her child, 32-year-old Gillian was noticed hammering the baby's head. 'It's the wrong shape. It's too long', she explained with no thought of the possible damage she may have incurred. As some would say, 'She's not in the same world as the rest of us.'

This is the type of postnatal illness with which psychiatrists are most familiar. They give sufferers immediate attention because they are so acutely ill. Most of the surveys on puerperal psychosis, studying the incidence, age, social class, and type of illness, have been undertaken by psychiatrists studying this type of hospital patient.

Usually there is an acute onset with a complete change of personality overnight. Indeed half of all psychotic patients are admitted within the first fourteen days after the birth. Many of them develop the illness immediately after labour as the following three women explain:

'After giving birth to both my babies I had the most horrific experience. A dreadful sinking sensation in which I had to fight very hard for control. It was as if I was being pulled down at very great speed.'

'The day after the Caesarean operation I woke up and the world looked different and smelt different. Horrible. I was swearing at everyone. Everyone was laughing at me and shouting obscenities. Men entered my room when they shouldn't be there.'

'I had to have an anaesthetic because the baby wasn't breathing well. The following day I was ill in the form of hearing imaginary voices talking to me. I was absolutely convinced of this and kept telling the nurses, of course no one believed me. After six days I was transferred to hospital and given treatment.'

Nurses in the postnatal ward are advised to keep a look out, for those mothers who appear agitated, over-active, interfering, complaining, over-demanding, suspicious, or tense. Also for those who are sure there's something wrong with their baby, or accuse the nurses of hurting or poisoning their child. These mothers may be in the early stages of a psychosis or it may be just a temporary phase due to the unfamiliar routine of hospital life. As already mentioned, such mothers who appear disturbed or unduly distressed in the first few days, may be advised to go home early in the hope that by returning to their own familiar surroundings their mental disturbance will subside, as indeed it sometimes does. However, if the mother continues with her abnormal behaviour then the general practitioner will be called in and he will either arrange direct admission to a mental ward, or will arrange a home visit by a consultant psychiatrist.

These ill patients are confused and muddled by bizarre thoughts, such as: 'I don't know which side is up' or one who described it as 'looking into a room in reverse'. If such patients are nursed at home it is essential for them to be under observation twenty-four hours of the day, every day, by their family or friends. Many have suicidal tendencies, and many of their actions are totally irrational; irreversible damage can occur very quickly while one's back is turned. Fortunately Hazel's baby avoided injury, although she confessed later:

'It was when baby Hugh looked up at me when I was breast-feeding. Those big blue eyes seemed to hypnotize me. I had a mad urge to stick a pin into those dark, black, circular pupils. Yes, it sounds unbelievable, but the strange urge was there and kept coming back. I loved the baby, yet felt absolutely murderous towards him.'

The patient lives in her own fantasy world removed from reality and unaware of her surroundings. She may have auditory hallucinations in which she hears voices, or visual hallucinations in which she sees imaginary people, animals, or things. She may have ruminating thoughts, during which she can't stop thinking about something, it keeps going round and round in her mind and she may ask the same question a dozen times over. Often there is some slight evidence of reality and word association, in which one word or the sight of one person triggers off a whole imaginary sequence. The next chapter, Nancy's Tale, provided by such a patient, admirably describes this type of irrational thought disorder.

Isobel, a 24-year-old mother, noticed a small pimple the size of a pinhead on her daughter's face when she was 2 days old. Isobel was in tears when she asked:

'Could it be a misplaced testes? Do you think Julie has spina bifida? Nobody tells the truth here, everyone is in conspiracy against me. They all say it's nothing, but it is something, I can see it.'

Dr Brockington and three other psychiatrists from the University Hospital of South Manchester studied twenty-six women admitted with puerperal psychosis and compared them with twenty-nine non-puerperal psychotic control women of the same ages and in the same hospital for similar symptoms. They noticed that their puerperal patients were more elated and sociable, but had lost less weight, were less angry and showed less verbal abuse than the control women. Most psychiatrists agree that puerperal women have a shorter stay in hospital compared with other women of the same age also suffering from psychosis.

Nature can be kind to such ill patients, for often they are left with no memory of those disturbing days. Karen wrote:

'There came a day a few weeks later when I could not remember what I had done for a whole week. They realized I was ill and I was admitted. I have had a loss of memory which means that I have forgotten a great deal about my first son's babyhood.'

But fortunately she has also forgotten the many strange, irrational acts which she committed during those missing days. This mother did not have ECT treatment while in hospital, but those who do receive it sometimes find there is a slight memory impairment later.

Patients with psychotic illnesses are admitted to hospital for their own safety. Increasingly nowadays there are facilities for the mother to be admitted with her new baby to a Mother and Baby Unit, where she can gradually become adjusted to her new baby, learn to care for him and also meet other mothers with their new babies. Gradually as they improve they are allowed home. Initially they go home for a few hours only, graduating to the weekend, and finally are fully discharged. However, on discharge these patients are not necessarily fully recovered, they are no longer a danger to themselves or to others, but they still need considerable support and help in caring for their baby, coping with a home and with the rest of the family. All too often the mothers are heavily tranquillized, slow, indecisive, and a mere shadow of their previous personality, with shuffling gait and expressionless faces, far removed from the alert, capable individuals of the prepregnancy era.

Dr Marvin Foundeur and his colleagues in New York followed up 100 patients with puerperal psychosis after a four-year interval and found three out of four had made 'a reasonable level of recovery', which is still a far cry from normality. In my experience the medication of many such patients masks the increase in symptoms, which occurs before menstruation. When patients try to reduce medication they notice an increase in symptoms within days or weeks and blame the reduction of medication for the increase of symptoms, without consideration of the day of the menstrual cycle. Such patients then return to their former heavy medication and it is a long time before they try to reduce again. If a patient has been on any medication for a time it will need to be reduced slowly over a matter of months, but the real answer is to keep a record of the severity of symptoms day by day in addition to noting the days of menstruation. (This is dealt with in Chapter 10.) If after two months the record shows a cyclical increase of symptoms around the time of menstruation, treatment with progesterone will remove the need for other medication with its tranquillizing action. A typical example is Lucy.

Lucy was 22 years of age when her daughter was born. Her pregnancy had been normal and the birth easy, but three days later it was noticed that she was deluded and she was found running down the hospital corridor crying and shouting 'Look, they've taken my baby away'. It was necessary to admit her to a local mental hospital, where she stayed for six months with occasional weekend leaves, and was eventually discharged, still taking drugs. Her husband noticed some years later that the days on which she deteriorated were the ten days before menstruation. She had not previously suffered from the premenstrual syndrome. When first seen, Lucy was heavily tranquillized on high doses of Stelazine (a major tranquillizer) and Fluanxol (a tricyclic antidepressant), and took no interest in her daughter, now 4½ years old, nor in her home. Her days were spent sitting about until her husband returned from work. She still had milk in both breasts. She was treated with progesterone from mid-cycle until menstruation, and over the following eight months her medication was very gradually withdrawn. Now she is alert and progressive, fully responsible in her shopping and housekeeping, and enjoying her daughter. Her only medication is progesterone for the second half of each menstrual cycle.

Thus treatment today can restore her to normal, but the psychosis, whilst it lasts is a very frightening and traumatic experience for all concerned. The next chapter deals with such a depression as experienced by Nancy, who wrote an account of how it all appeared to her. To quote her own words she wrote it to 'enlighten those who do not know what it is like to be "mentally ill", and to entreat them not to exhort those who are at the mercy of violent forces beyond their control to "pull yourself together" '. This account describes the torment of a muddled mind when it is forced beyond reality into imagination. It gives reasons for those episodes which cannot be explained by logical means, such as why she hid the apples, and the significance of putting the fruit bowl in the bath. It is a most revealing account which shows how a psychotic patient sometimes hears and sees people who are not there as well as smelling or tasting things which are not present. As we read Nancy's Tale we begin to realize that in mentally ill people all their five senses can be confused.

7
Nancy's tale

Nancy is 34 years old, a graduate in one of the top professions, who has continued her profession between her pregnancies. She had puerperal psychosis on four occasions, two so severe that she had to be hospitalized. During her last episode she responded dramatically to progesterone. This chapter is devoted entirely to her account of this illness, but names have been altered and a few lines omitted to preserve anonymity.

*

'Olivia's birth was a particularly traumatic one; she was in a breech position, so it was an emergency Caesarean, six and a half weeks early, my having had an internal haemorrhage, and Jason away in Edinburgh. Whilst waiting for the gynaecologist to arrive I had amused myself by reading a library book which gave an account of a supernatural visit to the author's Aunt by her dead cousin. Perhaps this affected me subconsciously – as the pre-med needle was inserted into the back of my hand I remonstrated jokingly with the anaesthetist that it was not one made by my husband's firm, but that of a competitor, but somewhere deep down I felt that there was just a chance that I would never wake up again. All I could think of to pray was: "Father, into thy hands I commend my spirit".

I believe there were six different drugs administered to me for the operation, some of them hallucinogenic. There was a whirling in my head. The spirits of my aborted baby and of my friend's miscarried baby were competing with a dark rush of wings to enter the body of my about-to-be-born baby. I definitely registered the moment that Olivia was born as a whiplash across my brain. Then I saw nothing. It wasn't that I *saw* nothing, but that in some way I seemed to utterly *understand* that nothing, and it was deeply, deeply terrifying. Normally one thinks of nothing as a space between two somethings, but this was not like that. It was a nothing so profound that it was not even an awareness of its own non-existence. I thought then that a knowing hell was greatly to be preferred to this ABSOLUTE non-existence. Pain – peace, pain – peace, life itself was a mere vibration of pain and peace, and the centre of the pendulum was rest, and rest was death. I became concerned that there was no wickedness left in the world, for how could positive (and it seems I identified myself with positive) exist in the absence of negative and still total nothing? My sister-in-law was with me when I came round, and can testify that I was greatly excited and disturbed.

After three weeks I returned home, leaving the baby still in hospital. I couldn't sleep, and I paced about all night. I had had the same reaction after the normal birth of my first child, ten days late, and so we were not unduly worried. That time it lasted about six weeks (as indeed it had the time before, when I had had an early abortion).

That Sunday evening a panel on the television were discussing the question of second marriage, and a saintly-looking Church of England monk was being asked his views. They were categorical. The church did not, and could never, approve second marriage. The sentence was final. God rejected me and I must go to hell, taking Jason with me. This programme was followed by a documentary about the Jewish religion.

That night I lay on the bed in my blue dressing-gown. I had insisted that Jason and I change places; he lay sleeping peacefully on my side of the bed, while I slept (I knew I *was* asleep) on his side on my back, like a living sacrifice on the pagan altar. The Rabbi stood at my bedside and leant over me. Unzipping my dressing-gown he opened up my body and looked into my soul.

"Where shall we begin?" I whispered to him.

"Let's start at Bethlehem", I heard him whisper in reply. (I have discovered how this was done – I whispered the words aloud myself, in my sleep.)

"That's funny", my whispers echoed, "My husband was born in Bethlehem!"

I woke up. I turned to look at Jason amazed. So he was Jesus Christ . . .

*

Jason was away and my mother came up to help out. She had brought some apples with her. Apples . . . the fall of man. Whatever happened we mustn't eat them, or we would be expelled from the Garden of Eden. Furtively I took them and frantically buried them, under the lilac tree in the furthermost right-hand corner of the back garden. I knew disaster to be overtaking us, and I cast about panic-stricken for the antidote. Death, opposite, life. So get the baby's carry-cot and put it in the right-hand corner of the sitting-room, diagonally opposite the apples, with Charles Dickens's *Great Expectations* in it.

*

I picked up the baby and went to my neighbour, who I knew had had three breakdowns. When I went out into the street the houses undulated. I thought that the end of the world would come down the street bouncing from side to side. Yes that was it, from Ken Lane at Number 33 to us at 22, then to Rita Simms at 44, and off to the Morrison's at No 11.

"Pam, I'm in a panic."

She got hold of her psychiatrist, to whom she managed to communicate some urgency, for he squeezed in an appointment for me two days later.

*

The disaster was the Flood, that was it. Jason was Noah. I ran up to the bathroom and filled the bath with water. I got the fruit bowl and floated it; in it I put Patrick's plastic farm animals, and a walnut. The nut was me; a nutcase, but also a tough nut to crack.

Jason was away in Italy. Something had happened to him, I was sure. Pam, my neighbour, took me to Heathrow Airport to meet him. The check-out point seemed to be in the bowels. (In fact it is at ground level but we had parked at first-floor level.) I was afraid to descend, everyone, including Pam, was smoking. I thought it was Hell, but I was determined to meet him, even if it meant descending into the jaws of Hell itself. The porters wore black uniforms with red bands round the caps and lapels. Yes,

Hell indeed, and they the Devil's agents . . . But he came through the barrier, surprised to see me, normal as ever . . .

*

Two other neighbours took me to the hospital. The baby had been taken back there as I was quite obviously not able to cope with her. I was convinced that she or I or both of us were about to die, or already dead. I was upset that she hadn't been christened, and wanted to arrange it immediately. Someone called sister. Sister looked dead white . . .

My neighbours (all true Samaritans indeed) took me on to my appointment with the psychiatrist. I was afraid of one of them (although she is actually one of the most likeable people I have ever met) – because she is barren. Sterility – the end of the world, no more life. I suffered for the other, for I felt her marriage to be imperfect.

"Are you happily married?" I asked her.

"Well, reasonably", she replied.

I mustn't get caught alone at the end of the world with a woman. If it was a man, we could have a baby, life could go on. Perhaps it was a trap and the psychiatrist was a woman? I refused to go in to see him. We stood on his doorstep in Harley Street and he came out to me. Deeply suspicious I refused to shake his hand.

"Hello", he said.

"Hello", I said, "how are you?" (He looked white, like sister had.)

"Oh, all right", he said, "except that I am worried about my investments now that the bottom appears to have fallen out of the property market." A property speculator! The Devil! I turned and fled. My neighbours chased me. I don't remember the journey home. One phoned my husband – the barren one. I wanted to get away from her.

Eventually Jason arrived, and took me home. I dressed all in white and insisted that he did the same. I was going to be properly married to him, in spite of being rejected by our church because of my having been married before. I went down to the kitchen. I would kill myself with the kitchen knife by plunging it into my heart. I got a red pencil and marked three crosses with it on my white dress over my heart.

My brother-in-law arrived. He was dressed in a blue shirt and blue jeans. But blue was the colour of the water, he would be drowned! He must be in white, the colour of the air! I wanted him to go home and change, but he wouldn't. (A superstition about this lingered, and to be on the safe side I gave him a white tie for a wedding present, as I told him, to keep his head above water when the time came.)

*

We were in a corridor, following a psychiatrist. He had a cigarette in his mouth.

"I don't think I like him", I said to Jason.

"Just go with him, he will look after you", Jason said.

"But he smokes!" I said.

"No I don't", he said and put the lighted cigarette in his pocket. (I asked him about this later. It wasn't a cigarette, it was a biro.)

I was met by a handsome coloured man.

"I'm glad it's you," I said, "because I believe in . . ."

"The brotherhood of man?" he asked.

"Yes, that's it" I said, and shook him warmly by the hand.

*

I woke up in a strange room, with no memories. I looked out of the window. The place looked like some kind of monastery (the Priory, Roehampton). So I WAS dead, after all! Heaven or Hell? Were the nurses angels or devils?

A special nurse was assigned to me, a Chinese girl called Sue. Oh NO! I was God and it was all my fault! If I was God, I would have power. To test my power, I threw my medicine in Sue's eyes. "Why did you do that?" asked Jason, who was standing by my bedside.

"Because I thought I was God."

*

The colour of the bedspread was of the greatest importance; I must get the sequence right. There was one on the bed and three more in the cupboard. Red: primeval, fire, etc. Brown: mud earth, life emerging. Blue next: sky, life, free, and then yellow: sun, ultimate release? I worked on it over and over.

*

I looked out of the window. There was Jason with his back to me, chatting to two people. He looked older. The baby had been brought to join me by this time. So she and I had died, and we had just waited here whilst the years went by, and finally Jason had died and come to join us. He was older than when I last saw him, but no matter, we were married and I loved him, I would go to him. I picked up the baby and walked out into the garden. When I drew near, they turned round. It wasn't Jason, it was a gardener. "Hello, do you want something?" I just walked away again.

*

My psychosis after Olivia was born was treated by electric shock, drug therapy, and psycho-analysis. I was advised not to have any more children, and it was six months before I began to feel like facing life again, and a year before I felt the return of my old energy and interest in life. For much of the time after I returned from hospital all I could do was sit apathetically on the sitting-room sofa. Even a visit from one of my best friends was a challenge for which I needed a stiff drink, and my hands trembled until she left.

When we discovered that I was pregnant again, the National Childbirth Trust put me in touch with an endocrinologist. I had intended that she should refer me to a psychiatrist who specialized in puerperal conditions, but she told me that there was no need. "You don't have a mental problem. You have a HORMONAL problem, and we will treat it with hormones."

It worked, and although I had to fight to hold on to my mind, and though I couldn't sleep and pushed my hospital bed to the window, gulping in the fresh air through the night and trying not to feel claustrophobic, my mind did not take off. Hormone injections were continued for about five weeks as far as I can recall, in fact, just longer than the date that the baby had been due. He was also early, this time by four weeks.

I breast-fed him for seven months, and why we did not realize that another hormone change would take place when he was weaned I'll never know. As it was, I dropped from five feeds to three in three days because I suddenly decided that the breast-feeding business had gone on too long. I immediately took off. I knew I was going under, and I kept meaning to tell Jason, but I kept fighting it, hoping to get over it, as I had done after the birth. Looking back I think this was due to a combination of pride, and fear of rejection. If it ever happens again I hope that I will have sufficient humility, and sufficient trust in the compassion of others, to seek help earlier.

Just before I cracked up completely we went to a "Masked Ball" at the Hurlingham Club. I was experiencing that growing feeling of imminent danger, although it was still under control. Jason was in his white dinner jacket (symbolizing Jesus Christ again), and before entering I was given a red mask. I almost refused it, for it made me look diabolic, until I realized the logic of it. God and the Devil, the ultimate and only indissoluble marriage, the one calling into existence the other. I felt that we would be safe together. There was some mix-up over the tables, and we were shown to table eleven (eleven, worshipped by some tribal religions as a number with mystical powers), and the man who was double-booked for table eleven – a MR SLAUGHTER – was shown elsewhere. So we were to escape slaughter, after all. (Who can say that there was not some divine sense of humour behind that coincidence?)

The final collapse was triggered by the penultimate episode of Dickens's *Our Mutual Friend* on television. When the odious schoolteacher attacked the young hero his screams seemed to go right through me to the marrow of my bones. Lizzie stood rooted to the spot. "Why doesn't she go to him, why doesn't she help him?" I ask Jason.

"She's paralysed with fear."

That night as I lay asleep I was in the grip of terrible dreams. I was given three eggs from the fridge (my three children). Which came first, the chicken or the egg? Human flesh, it tastes like chicken, the end of the world, everyone was rushing after each other to eat them, no, no, hide, under the table, no, rush into the open countryside, listen, you and I will stay together, I won't eat you if you won't eat me, here we are helping each other out of reach of those ravenous mouths, no, NO, they've got my feet (I struggled to free my feet and legs under the blankets). NO! NO! I was screaming, but no sound was coming out. I was paralysed. Jason lay beside me with his back to me. Why doesn't he help me? Because he's asleep, and anyway he can't hear you. Then I felt the sands rushing off me from the mid-line, and I seemed to come back up into my body from below, like coming up from out of the grave.

CRACK, CRACK, CRACK. Someone outside just above the road on the opposite side was being whipped with incredible ferocity. I counted thirty lashes. So it was Jesus Christ again.

"Alright, alright, I forgive myself, only please," I pleaded, "please don't ask me to live without you!"

I was flung back into my body with abrupt contempt. I woke up in my body, sweating. Without who? What had happened? I was sobbing, but I felt some sort of relief, some sort of completion. I looked at Jason beside me. It seemed that all I wanted was to be allowed to be with him. "Don't ask me to live without you". Yes, I would be alright so long as he was there.

The next day Jason went to Italy. While he was away I felt an absolute compulsion to get to the bottom of "What it's all about". I read *The Book on the Taboo Against Knowing Who You Are*, and when he returned the psychosis had gone too far for prevention. I tried to explain. "I know the TRUTH", I sobbed.

"What truth?"

"There's only one of us here. You are me and I am you. Self is everywhere, there's no escape from it, only Self, whichever way you turn." He rang the doctor.

There were voices in my head. One sobbed and pleaded and seemed to be growing its way up the inside of the back of my head. The other encouraged and comforted and seemed to be seeing the sobbing one through the ordeal. I told the doctor only about the sobbing one, though. It said "Mummy, Mummy, you said you were going to look after me, and you're letting them eat me!"

I was immediately admitted to the Psychiatric Unit at St Mary's Hospital.

Jason and the endocrinologist had a terrific fight to get the hospital to agree to give me hormone injections. Even when they reluctantly agreed to do so it was in conjunction with their own drug therapy. The hormone supplies took three days to get hold of. Once injections were started I got well so rapidly that everyone was astonished. I was discharged after two weeks without medication, and returned to work after a further week feeling NORMAL. Energy, normal. Thoughts, normal. Libido, normal. Contrast this with the six months to one year that it took me to get over the first episode.

While I was in hospital I saw two things which could not, in reality as we think we know it, have been there. The first was Jason. He was in the next ward, and waved cheerfully to me as he disappeared out of sight round a corner. I struggled with the nurses to be allowed to go after him, and made such a fuss that I was taken through the double-doors into the next ward to be shown that he was not there, and that he was at work, and would visit me at visiting time.

The other was two suns in the sky. I stood at the window and watched them, fascinated, knowing that the end of the world would come when they merged. (Did they or not? I don't know.)

The most disturbing things that can't be explained were the voices outside the window which cried softly "NO! NO!"

*

Ultimate pain, or ultimate ecstasy? I wasn't sure. And the SMELL. I kept BUMPING INTO it. It smelt like cauterized flesh. I always drew back, immediately, but it seemed to hem me in. I was afraid that I was burning someone when I bumped into it. I always asked a nurse: "That SMELL! What is it?" and they always replied "What smell? I can't smell anything."

On about the second day, as I sat in the canteen bewildered and terrified, one of the waiters came up to me and muttered:

"Your God is behind you, your God is beside you, your God is in front of you, have no fear."

God bless you, Spanish waiter, wherever you are, for those

words! They were something to hold on to, and gave me hope.

I lay on my bed, and my head and my body were two different people. My body was totally relaxed. (The drugs?) My head seemed to be in direct communication with the sun, and all it said was:

"The will to live, the will to live, the will to live . . ."

As I lay there, something fluttered in my body, it beat against its prison, and tried to get out. Now it was over my stomach, now my shoulder, now under my right breast. INSIDE ME, a cock crowed three times (so Peter had betrayed Christ) and my flesh jumped where it crowed. (Muscles twitching? Stomach gurgling?) Suddenly a switch was turned off in my head, just "Flick!" like that, and I got up. Whatever that was in my body it was going to rush up through my mouth and pull me inside-out. I must keep it down, at all costs! I began to strangle myself with my belt. The nurse rushed up alarmed, and tried to stop me ("You're hurting yourself!"), but it subsided and I let go. My face felt all red, but my head and my body were still different beings, and my body felt fine. (Question: Do your insides feel as though they are corroding? How did you know that Professor Priest? I'll not give in to *that* and admit it!)

I thought they were holding Jason and I apart, and that something terrible was happening to him and the children. I began to plot my escape. I took a pillow and tried to smash the window. (Armour-plated glass.) Then I borrowed Sue's scissors and tried to unscrew the window. Hopeless. So I took a wire coat-hanger, and holding it like a hook, determined to fight my way out. The first nurse who saw me with it took it off me (I couldn't bring myself to use it, after all). So I decided that the only thing to do was to use my wits. The staff nurse on duty was coloured. I started to shout at him. "You let me out of here! I have a doll at home, *you* know what I mean, and I'm going to stick a pin in its THROAT! I am the one with the POWER! And when I get up there, I'm going to tell on YOU, I'm going to tell them that you won't let me OUT!"

A whole group of nurses were clucking round me (just like hens, I thought). They seemed afraid to touch me, but eventually they started bundling me back into my room. (One coloured mammy-looking nurse, especially, kept muttering: "HUH! Jus' who does she think she IS?" and days later, when I passed her, she said to one of the other nurses: "Huh! She oughta wash herself, get rid of de STINK!" which, as I was regaining my senses by that time, amused me in a surprised way.)

A very nice young lady doctor arrived, and she was really sweating.

"Why are you afraid of me?" I asked her.

Like a cornered animal I stood up on my bed and contemplated trying to strangle her with her gold necklace, but I hadn't the heart to do it, besides which it was futile, I was outnumbered.

"You want to hurt me! You are going to do something to me!"

"No, I'm not, I'm just going to give you an injection to calm you down, it won't hurt, it's just a little prick . . ."

I was in the road, with no slippers on, just my nightie. It was cold. I saw a lorry with some sacks in it, and I thought if I got into one and hopped along it would keep my feet warm. I seemed to float effortlessly up into the lorry and got the sack. I started to hobble along in it. A breakdown lorry came along pulling a car. I stopped the man.

"You've got to help me, please, take me home to my husband . . ."

"Well, I don't know love, you'll have to ask the Guvnor 'ere, 'e's in charge." They moved off, but then it seemed to happen again, and they were back.

Of course, this sounds like a dream, but it really did happen, I really did escape from the hospital into the road. No one knows how I managed it, full of Valium and who knows what else, but there were the brown stains from the sacking on the soles of my feet to prove it.

I thought that the hospital was electrically charged, and indeed, there must be considerable static in there from all those electric shocks that they give people, and from those relentless floor polishers that are given free reign every day to terrify the germs. When in the reception area my head really buzzed with disturbance, which it seemed to receive from all over the place. I spilt some water on my canvas shoe and it seemed to take up electricity into the ball of my foot. (Actually, with hindsight, I think it gave me rheumatism.)

More voices. Again one was sobbing (this time with remorse) and one comforting. The sobbing one I identified with myself, the comforting one with Jason. Whether the conversations really took place, or whether they were just in my head, I do not know, all I know is that there, at the bottom of the pit, I found perfect comfort and understanding. I think he really was there when I said: "I feel that I have a duty to kill myself", and he replied: "Well, all I can do, darling, is to ask you, with great humility, not to do it. The children and I need you . . ."

*

My recovery was swift and total, and our ardent prayer is that we will never have to go through all that again! I shall never forget the way Jason looked at the end of that two weeks, when he brought the baby up to see me. He looked as though he had spent his last ounce of strength to reach the top step, and was about to collapse.'

*

Nancy's Tale is a shattering account of her experience of an illness which fortunately is rare. It shows the effect upon her husband, whose behaviour throughout fills one with admiration. A most satisfactory detail of the story not only for Nancy but also for future potential sufferers, is that once progesterone treatment was underway "recovery was swift and beautiful".

We now go on to deal with a hidden disaster which often follows depression but which is not necessarily the result of postnatal depression. The loss of sexual desire is of great importance to the future happiness of husbands and wives.

8
Not tonight, darling

A similar remark – 'Not tonight, Josephine' – was attributed to Napoleon, and has been considered a classical rejection of nocturnal sexual pleasure. If we can believe all the accounts Napoleon had good reasons for his desire to abstain. They were, however, very different from those that are considered here.

Fully satisfying sexual activity has been described as 'the cement of a good marriage', and while it is accepted that a happy marriage can exist without sexual activity there is no escaping the fact that complete sexual satisfaction strengthens and enriches the marriage bond between husband and wife, weaving strong ties of trust and faithfulness within marriage. Both partners need the contentment and full relaxation that true sexual enjoyment brings.

One of the problems that childbirth can produce in the mother is a loss of sexual pleasure and desire, or loss of libido, while the husband still keenly desires his sexual activity. This loss of interest can be the result of postnatal depression. It can, however, also arise from causes unrelated to postnatal depression and so the subject is dealt with separately in this chapter.

For many wives the greatest possible insult is for the husband to refer to her as 'frigid' or 'ice cold'. Yet there are many different degrees of loss of sexual desire such as the woman who recoils the moment she hears her husband's key go into the lock of the front door or as he advances across the lounge. Some women will even object to a mere peck on the cheek, or an arm around the shoulder or waist and will make it quite obvious that there are no opportunities as yet for any sexual activity. Then there are other women who fully enjoy the kisses, caresses, cuddles, and love-play beforehand, but unrealistically would like it all to stop there. Possibly they are frightened of any pain that may be caused or they may feel quite unable to face up to the frustration that a lack of climax or orgasm may bring.

Doctors and marriage guidance counsellors frequently hear the statement 'Libido is non-existent now', and 'We've had no sex since the last baby was born'. This loss of libido is not found by the obstetrician for the same reason that he may miss the postnatal depression. His postnatal examination is performed before sexual activity has been resumed or postnatal depression has become apparent. Many books about having a baby suggest that sexual activities should not be enjoyed until after the postnatal examination, so that brings it out of the obstetrician's responsibility. The loss is frequently reported to the family doctor some months after the baby's birth, he may then attempt some treatment before calling in a psychiatrist, and so quite a long time may elapse after the onset, before the woman meets the psychiatrist. The psychiatrist is seeing the woman too late for a quick resolution of her problems and his task is therefore much more difficult.

Where there was complete sexual fulfilment before the pregnancy, the cause for the loss of libido after the birth of the child can come under one of four headings: postnatal depression, psychological, hormonal, and structural.

Postnatal depression

Loss of libido is one of the recognized losses that can occur in the disease of loss, or depression, be it the typical depressive illness or postnatal depression. It is a symptom which disappears when the depression passes. Even those who are only affected with mild postnatal exhaustion, without marked depression, may find they are too tired to be aroused. Two husbands explained:

'Marion falls asleep easily in the day and is always in bed – she is floating on a cloud of her own and sex is dead."
'Pat can't make love and is generally sunk in a slough of misery, which pervades her whole life and that of everyone around her.'

In the confused state of her postnatal depression Rosalind

noticed: 'It is when my sex urge is greatest that I refuse my husband and find an outlet in some impossible affair.'

Treatment of depression with some antidepressants may also cause loss of sex interest, though fortunately if the cause of the sexual problem is depression there will be a return to full sexual desire and arousal once the depression lifts.

Psychological causes

The sexual desires may already have diminished in the early weeks of pregnancy, especially if the child is unwanted and there are any thoughts or discussions on the possibility of terminating the pregnancy. Again the presence of symptoms of early pregnancy, such as morning sickness, depression, tiredness, or headaches, may decrease sexual interest. Occasionally when there has been a previous difficulty in conception, a history of previous miscarriages, actual or threatened, or unexpected bleeding in the first weeks, the couple may have been advised to abstain during the early months of pregnancy. Many a couple take this advice too seriously and go on to abstain throughout the full nine months. Others find the alteration in the woman's shape in pregnancy a hindrance to their normal position for intercourse, and instead of trying another position they will abstain until the end of pregnancy. When there has been a considerable period of abstention the resumption of sexual activity may be deferred long after the original cause has ended.

There are those women who found the pregnancy difficult or the labour horrifying and they are determined not to start another pregnancy, 'never – no – never'. They may claim that during their hospital stay they chatted with women who were pregnant in spite of good contraceptives being used. These women need help in building up their confidence with some other contraceptive method. However, it is never wise to sterilize one of the partners permanently in the hope that sex interest will return once the fear of pregnancy has been permanently abolished. There may be other causes for the loss of libido which remain untouched and which do not need such drastic, irreversible measures.

There may be jealousy over the baby, the woman feeling that too much of her time or too much of her husband's interest is devoted to the little one. She may be suspicious that while she was away in hospital having the baby her husband was out having an affair.

Hormonal causes

At the time of the birth of the baby there are tremendous and sudden changes in the level of the mother's hormones. Her body is called upon to adapt to these altered amounts of chemicals flowing in her blood, and sometimes there is difficulty with this adaptation. This is particularly so in respect of the hormones prolactin, oestrogen, progesterone, and testosterone. All of these are involved in the creation of sexual desire. It has already been mentioned that when breast-feeding has stopped, the hormone prolactin should normally reduce to its pre-pregnancy level. However, when this is still raised after breast-feeding has ended it results in a marked loss of desire. Fortunately this raised level of prolactin can easily be recognized by a blood test, and be corrected by giving one or two tablets daily of bromocriptine. In these cases the bromocriptine is remarkably effective in restoring the normal sexual desires within a matter of weeks. Indeed a temporary excessive desire may be experienced, until the hormone balance returns to normal control. Less frequently the fault lies in abnormal levels of oestrogen or progesterone and these can be correctly balanced by administration of the appropriate hormone.

Sometimes the hormones in the Pill are responsible for upsetting the normal hormone balance of the body and may cause a loss of libido. Fortunately if this is the cause it is easily remedied and some other form of contraceptive chosen.

Structural changes

After her first child, Sheila asked:

'Why, after waiting nine months and receiving such a wonderful reward, am I not ready for sex? Has my vagina altered? Why have I changed?'

The answer here is that a considerable number of alterations take place in the vagina during the birth process. To fully understand these changes it is easier to first consider the alterations which occur in the vagina during orgasm. A normal vagina is a straight passage leading from the outside to the door of the womb or cervix, and it is into the vagina that the penis is inserted during intercourse. During intercourse with orgasm there is a throbbing of the upper end of the vagina, which dilates, and there is a constriction of the lower end of the vagina.

Now consider the changes which occur during labour in a normal vaginal delivery. Gradually with the contractions of the womb the cervix opens. Whereas before labour the cervix could barely admit a drinking straw, during labour it stretches and opens wide enough to allow a baby's head, with a diameter of about 10 centimetres (4 inches), to pass through, and the vagina as such disappears (Figures 3 and 4). If the baby's head comes out

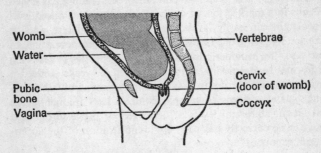

Fig. 3. The baby's head before labour

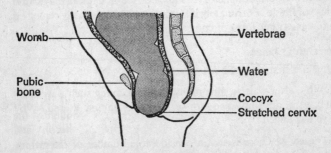

Fig. 4. The baby's head just before birth

suddenly with a marked propulsive force there may be a tear of the skin or vaginal wall. There is invariably a tear in the cervix, even in an apparently normal delivery, but this does not need any stitches.

The mechanism of childbirth is remarkable and within a very short time the anatomy is restored, the cervix contracts, and the womb, which once held the baby as well as the waters and placenta, shrinks down within six weeks to almost, but never quite, its pre-pregnancy size.

This is what happens in a normal vaginal delivery, but there are instances when nature alone does not complete the job and perhaps instruments, or forceps, are required to lift out baby's head, or there may be a tear which has to be stitched. The site where the stitches are may become inflamed or even infected, and they are painful. Birth is a traumatic process with massive changes in size and position of these organs, and sometimes when it is all finished it is possible that the nerves which come into action in orgasm are injured, either permanently or they may take a long time to heal. Where this is suspected as the cause for the loss of desire the woman should be advised to resume normal activities to allow healing to be expedited.

In other cases women may experience pain at intercourse, when previous to pregnancy it has been painfree. Where this is pain on entry it can be due to painful stitches because the stitching has made the entrance too small or too rigid, so that it won't stretch. This is only a temporary difficulty and will soon resolve with normal sexual activity. Sometimes the pain may arise from the very fear that entry will be painful.

Pain on thrusting may result from infection, either in the pelvic floor, in the bladder, or vagina. It needs a full gynaecological examination to decide what the problem is, but once the source of infection is treated the pain disappears.

There are women who claim that the tingling effect of some effervescent contraceptive pessaries helps to encourage sexual pleasure. It is a simple tip and well worth trying. Loss of sexual desire is a tragedy in a woman who previously had full enjoyment. If it occurs following childbirth it should be investigated and treated – the sooner the better.

9
Who is at risk?

'Novelists tell us that women blossom and exude happiness and vitality in pregnancy – do they?'

This question was asked by a highly respected psychiatrist at a medical luncheon in the North Middlesex Hospital, London, on a summer's day in 1965. It provoked a heated discussion: 'Of course they do!' – 'Certainly the majority of women have increased vitality at this time' asserted the general practitioner obstetricians. 'I never meet them' retorted the psychiatrist and his colleagues.

Out of that exchange of views arose a research project that was to provide all of them with a better understanding of the emotional changes of pregnancy and the puerperium. A group of fourteen – general practitioner obstetricians and a psychiatrist – joined forces to discover exactly what were the characteristics of those women who blossomed in pregnancy. Obviously, such women would have no cause to see a psychiatrist, so why did he ask that question? For many of those doctors present this was the introduction to a new interest in postnatal depression.

There and then each general practitioner obstetrician agreed to fill in a special form for each patient at their routine antenatal examinations. This form would provide details of age, occupation, general health, and previous psychiatric breakdowns in patient and family; it would state whether she was placid, normal, or anxious. Another form was also filled in with the usual antenatal details of weight, blood pressure, urine test, and so on. As soon as they were completed the forms were posted off to a special research secretary at the hospital. This was to ensure that the doctor would not refer to them at the next antenatal visit. 500 women were initially entered into the scheme and all particulars were duly recorded at their monthly, and later weekly, antenatal visits and then, after the baby was born, at their sixth-day, sixth-week, and sixth-month postnatal visits.

At the end, all the forms were carefully compared and studied and it was found that 7 per cent of the mothers had developed postnatal depression severe enough to need medical treatment, although none of them required admission to hospital. In other parts of the world doctors had studied different aspects of these problems and their findings were in complete agreement with the findings of the North Middlesex work, which emphasized the characteristics of the women who were at risk of developing post-natal depression. What were those characteristics? 'The women who blossom and exude happiness and vitality in pregnancy!'

The survey showed that it was just those women who were happiest, elated, and euphoric during the later months of their pregnancies who were at risk, for 64 per cent of them developed postnatal depression compared with 24 per cent of the other women. The mothers developing postnatal depression had two outstanding characteristics: a favourable attitude to motherhood, and labile emotions (unstable emotions, liable to change). They were the ones who welcomed pregnancy, were happy and elated during pregnancy, and with few of those annoying pregnancy symptoms like depression, irritability, tiredness, sickness, back-ache, and headache. When they were asked during the last month of pregnancy whether they wished to breast-feed they answered with a resounding 'Yes'. But they did have their mood swings, being more anxious at the first interview, elated during the preg-nancy, and then depressed after the birth. The majority of medical papers and textbooks dealing with postnatal depression assume that it has a psychological explanation but many of the findings of the survey, especially the findings of marked maternal charac-teristics and labile emotions, tend to diminish the psychological in favour of a hormonal explanation (more about that in Chapter 12).

There were other important findings in the survey, which would also appear to weigh against a psychological explanation. The women who developed postnatal depression had no higher inci-dence of previous psychiatric illness or of psychiatric illness in their families than did normal women. There was no difference between those who had difficult deliveries and those with easy ones, nor in those who had abnormal babies, and those who had healthy ones. Again this confirmed the findings of other workers. Dr Mary Martin, at the Rotunda Hospital in Dublin, found that postnatal depression was not related to the length of labour, the difficulty of labour, a forceps delivery, or the incidence of pre-eclampsia (PE). Neither was it related to high blood pressure in pregnancy, nausea and vomiting in pregnancy, age, or marital status; nor with failure to breast-feed.

The effect of stillbirth

The *Lancet* in 1979 carried a report by Dr Michael Clarke and Dr Anthony Williams of a study of two groups of 300 women living in Leicestershire. In one group of mothers the baby had been stillborn or had died within seven days of birth, in the other group the mothers all had healthy, normal babies. They reported that postnatal depression was more marked in younger mothers of 24 years and under, and among these mothers the incidence of postnatal depression at six months after the birth was the same for the mothers with healthy babies as for those mothers who had lost their babies. They also estimated from their survey that in England and Wales there must be some 23,000 women annually who are at least moderately depressed within six months of their baby's birth.

A personal study

To study the characteristics of those who develop postnatal depression, and particularly to find the incidence of recurrence in subsequent pregnancies the author scrutinized the medical records in her own practice and in her hospital clinic, of all women who had suffered from postnatal depression during the last ten years and had been seen by her personally. This is probably the largest series of patients with postnatal depression personally studied by one doctor. Most of such studies in medical literature have resulted from a search of hospital records of patients with the severe form of puerperal psychosis, who have been seen by numerous other doctors with varying definitions and standards. This personal study was limited to married women, who had suffered their first psychiatric illness within six months of a full-term pregnancy and which required medical treatment. The survey covered 413 women of whom 217 (53 per cent) had only required treatment from their general practitioner and so were classified as 'mild'; 113 women (27 per cent) had needed treatment from a psychiatrist and were classified as having an illness of 'moderate' severity; and eighty-three (20 per cent) had suffered from psychosis requiring hospital admission and were classified as 'severe'.

Possibility of recurrence

The 413 women had a total of 915 full-term pregnancies among which were eighty-eight women who had only one affected pregnancy (many women said that they had been advised to have no further pregnancies because of the risk of a return of their psychiatric illness). There were a further 104 women who had more than one child but had had no further pregnancy following the one after which they had suffered a postnatal breakdown. This left 221 women who had a subsequent pregnancy after the affected pregnancy, and among these women as many as two-

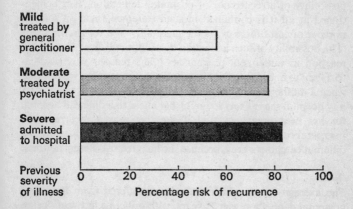

Fig. 5. Risk of recurrence of postnatal depression in subsequent pregnancy (221 pregnancies)

thirds (68 per cent) had another postnatal depression. Sometimes the second illness was worse than the first, and in others it was of the same severity or not quite so bad, but in every case it was bad enough to require further medical treatment. Furthermore of those with the severe form of psychosis over 84 per cent had a recurrence (Figure 5).

However, the recurrence rate was not 100 per cent and there seemed to be no way in which a recurrence could be predicted. The survey included five women, each of whom had six normal pregnancies with normal labours, and each time with the delivery of a healthy child. One woman developed postnatal depression after every pregnancy, another developed it after each of her first four pregnancies, another had it after each of her first three pregnancies, another had it after her second and fourth only, and the other woman had it only after her last pregnancy (Figure 6). Mathematicians will tell us that we have not exhausted all the possible combinations and permutations for a woman having postnatal depression following one or more of her six pregnancies. So it seems there is no way of telling what the outcome might be.

The current textbooks on psychiatry are rather vague about the possibility of a recurrence of postnatal depression. If it is mentioned at all it is contained in such statements as: 'In a small number of cases there exists the possibility of a recurrence' and: 'The possibility of such a reaction does not predispose to a similar reaction in subsequent pregnancies.' The reasons why psychiatrists fail to appreciate the high recurrence rate might well be that when a mother has had the unfortunate experience in one maternity hospital she is likely to go further afield to a different hospital for her next pregnancy and if she then has a recurrence of puerperal psychosis she will be referred to a psychiatric ward in a different catchment area, because she has given a different address.

Age

The average age at which the women suffered from their first postnatal depression was 26 years, with only one in twenty being outside the range 21–31 years. Further analysis showed the chances of developing postnatal depression was not related to the

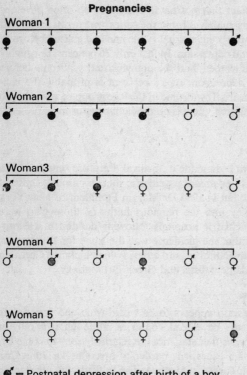

Pregnancies

Woman 1

Woman 2

Woman3

Woman 4

Woman 5

♂ = Postnatal depression after birth of a boy
♂ = Normal puerperium after birth of a boy
♀ = Postnatal depression after birth of a girl
♀ = Normal puerperium after birth of a girl

Fig. 6. Occurrence of postnatal depression in five women, who each had six pregnancies

age at the first pregnancy, the interval between pregnancies, whether under two years or over ten years, or to the sex of the child.

The premenstrual syndrome

In view of the fact that postnatal depression so often develops into the premenstrual syndrome the series was further analysed to find whether the premenstrual syndrome had started before or after the postnatal depression. In fact only 26 per cent, or roughly a quarter of the women, had the premenstrual syndrome before their postnatal depression. As 26 per cent is probably the incidence of premenstrual syndrome in this age group of women who have not had children, there is no predictive factor in its presence or absence.

Religious factors

Suggestions have been made in medical literature that there is a high incidence of postnatal psychiatric illnesses among those of the Jewish faith, but in 1956 Dr Marvin Foundeur of New York reported a survey into the religious faiths of those who were admitted to psychiatric hospitals following childbirth. He produced evidence that the incidence was the same for Protestants, Jewesses, Roman Catholics, and others (which included Christian Scientists, Fundamentalists, and Greek Orthodox).

Primitive peoples

Postnatal depression appears to be world-wide and is certainly not limited to the developed countries, although it is only in developed countries that statistics are relatively easy to come by. In some primitive tribes it is harder to assess as Dr John Cox discovered in his survey in Uganda. The difficulty was in finding suitable non-pregnant control women in a culture where it is a stigma for a woman to be either single or infertile. Nevertheless Dr Cox did find an incidence of 9·7 per cent of postnatal depression among 186 Ganda women attending an antenatal clinic in a semi-rural health centre. This is remarkably similar to the incidence of 10 per cent found by Dr Brice Pitt in his study of women attending the antenatal clinic of the London Hospital.

Dr Brazelton of Harvard studied women in Guatemala and Sumatra and also found postnatal depression in these primitive tribes. He sees it as a force for doing good – a counterbalance to the physical and psychological tension built up during pregnancy. He suggests that postnatal depression is a way of telling the mother to slow down so she can gather the energy needed for looking after the new baby.

Jean Liedloff, an anthropologist, who has studied a Stone Age tribe in Venezuela, recalled the absence of postnatal depression, which she attributed to the fact that they did not separate the baby from the mother immediately after birth. However, two distinguished anthropologists, Margaret Mead, now based in New York, and Professor Jean la Fontaine, of the London School of Economics, both doubt whether anthropologists have the necessary medical or psychological expertise to detect postnatal depression in primitive cultures. They both disagree with the simplistic view that 'back to nature' automatically means all goes well in motherhood; 'doing what comes naturally' may mean that scores of women die in childbirth.

Dr Pitt agrees that contact with the mother immediately after birth does have an effect on the mother's behaviour towards the baby and on breast-feeding, but he doubts whether removal of the baby immediately after birth has the effect of causing post-natal depression which may begin many weeks later. In home confinements in England the mother is usually given the baby to hold immediately after delivery, not so much to encourage pair bonding as to give the midwife some valuable extra minutes to get on with the many other jobs which need doing after delivery, but the incidence of postnatal depression is the same in home deliveries as in hospital deliveries.

Genetic influence

The influence of a genetic factor in depression is being widely appreciated and there does appear to be a genetically inherited factor in postnatal depression in the same way that some families are more prone to develop a depressive illness than others, but this is not the major causative factor. Two examples are Sandra and Tracy. Sandra was admitted to a mental hospital after the birth of her daughter Jane and was discharged after an interval of thirty years. Jane had four pregnancies, two requiring admission for puerperal psychosis, and the third was followed by postnatal depression treated by a psychiatrist. Jane received prophylatic progesterone therapy for her fourth pregnancy and was well throughout the postnatal period.

Tracy's husband had been admitted for depression before her marriage. She had five children and developed puerperal psychosis on each occasion. Her three sons and three grandsons all had a depressive illness between the ages of 20 and 32 years, and both daughters and one granddaughter had puerperal psychosis. One granddaughter escaped depression because she never became pregnant.

Post-abortal psychosis

In Sweden Dr Jansson noted that psychosis was more common after a full-term pregnancy than after an abortion, and that post-abortal depression was especially common in those who had previously suffered a puerperal psychosis. In Britain women who have a termination of pregnancy may feel some measure of guilt, and so do not easily seek help for their depression, feeling that they have brought it on themselves, and if they ask for medical help some months later they are apt to 'forget' the incident at their first interview. As a result figures for the incidence of post-abortal depression in Britain are only possible in respect of those whose illness was so severe that admission to hospital was required.

Adoption

Depression can occur among adoptive mothers and fathers during the first six months after they receive their adopted child. However, the incidence of depression in adoptive parents is no greater than in the normal population. Psychiatrists are apt to blame the puerperal breakdown on the hazards associated with the new baby's arrival, but the fact that adoptive parents are no more prone to depression than non-adoptive adults, suggests that it cannot fairly be blamed on such superficial factors as disturbed sleep produced by the baby crying, the increased work and responsibility that a baby brings, or the divided love of the husband for the child and wife. Furthermore the illness in an adoptive mother is typical depression rather than the atypical type of postnatal depression.

Infertility

Dr C N Naylor of the Central Middlesex Hospital, London, produced evidence to show that postnatal depression is more common among those who have been trying to conceive for longer than two years. The question is often asked 'What accounts for the apparent rise in the incidence of postnatal depression?' Well, we really don't know whether there has been a rise in incidence. It could be that diagnosis has improved and it is being recognized more easily, possibly mothers are becoming more eager to ask for treatment at an earlier stage. If there is a raised incidence it could be related to the widespread use of hormonal contraceptives. It has also been suggested that the greater use of drugs to accelerate the birth process is responsible. There is the possibility that the use of drugs and hormones to assist conception play a part. The simple answer is that we really do not know. However, we do know the frequency with which the various forms occur as shown in Figure 7.

Many factors have been considered in this chapter to enable us

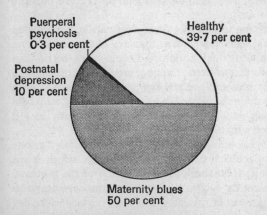

Fig. 7. Frequency of postnatal illnesses

to recognize the pregnant mother who is likely to have a psychiatric illness after the birth of her child. But apart from a history of a previous postnatal depression, there are at present no other indications to enable us to make a definite prediction. There is certainly a need for wider education on the subject in medical circles, as is shown by the North Middlesex Hospital Survey. When the interviews were all finished, and before the doctors who had been participating began to analyse the forms, it was decided to invite the other doctors who frequented the lunch meetings to join us in answering a questionnaire of some twenty questions, requiring Yes/No answers, on what they thought would be the findings of the survey. There were fifty doctors of all ranks from elderly consultants to newly qualified housemen who agreed to try. They were general practitioners, obstetricians, community physicians, and psychiatrists. The results were an eye opener for they got only 38 per cent of the answers correct. Had it been a real examination they would all have failed! Only one doctor correctly forecast that women with the fewest symptoms in pregnancy would be most likely to develop postnatal depression. Most doctors seemed to expect that their usual problem patients, such as the women with a previous or family history of psychiatric illness or women with many pregnancy symptoms, would be problem patients in the postnatal period. The opposite was correct.

It was interesting to find that those doctors who participated in the survey did significantly better than any of the others; those with higher obstetric qualifications did significantly better than those without further obstetric training; general practitioners did better than the obstetricians and the psychiatrist; and women readers will no doubt be pleased to learn that women doctors did better than their male colleagues, but not significantly so – it could have been a matter of chance!

This emphasizes once again the need for more education among doctors on the problem of postnatal depression, which is the most common and most serious complication of the postnatal period. At present the subject receives only scant coverage in an textbook of obstetrics or psychiatry; we look forward to the day when it receives full coverage in textbooks of both specialities.

10
There's a time for everything

There is a time which clearly determines the difference between typical depression and postnatal depression, and that is the puerperium, which is subject to a legal definition.

In England and Wales the puerperium is defined as the fourteen days after a woman has given birth to a child, while in Scotland the puerperium lasts twenty-one days.

Maternity blues

The mildest form of postnatal depression is the maternity blues which develops during the third to eighth day after the birth of the baby. As already explained it is a relatively short-lived phenomenon and is usually all over by the end of the first two weeks. In the early part of this century it was usual for the patients to be kept in hospital for the full fourteen days after the birth to help the mother overcome any emotional problems, but today many women are discharged after twenty-four or forty-eight hours and are then cared for at home by a midwife.

Postnatal exhaustion

Postnatal exhaustion has a slow onset, beginning either directly after the birth or developing slowly during the first month or six weeks. It lingers on for six to nine months and has usually disappeared after the baby's first birthday. Mothers whose energy does not return to normal naturally are the ones who are likely to develop postnatal depression, and later the premenstrual syndrome.

Postnatal depression

Postnatal depression may start at the birth, following on as a continuation of maternity blues, in which case involuntary tears will give way to a general sadness and other symptoms of depression. For some women it does not start immediately, and they have a few weeks or months feeling exhilarated and congratulating themselves on their good fortune before the depression sets in. The later onset may be associated with the stopping of breast-feeding, although in other women the depression ends as they finish breast-feeding. The depression may accompany the first premenstruum (the days immediately before menstruation) after birth and then continue with increasing severity during each subsequent menstruation. Sometimes it starts when the mother first returns to the contraceptive pill, especially the progestogen-only type. The mother has usually been taking the Pill without any side effects, but she does not appreciate that the hormonal upheaval of pregnancy and labour may have played havoc with her hormone balance, and so she joins the ranks of those who, because of side effects, are no longer able to tolerate the Pill.

Puerperal psychosis

Those unfortunate women who are prone to puerperal psychosis will often find the onset is immediately they return from the labour ward or shortly afterwards. In fact, half of all women admitted to hospital with puerperal psychosis have an onset of illness within two weeks of the birth. Dr Foundeur, in a study of women with puerperal psychosis and women of the same ages with psychosis not related to childbirth, noted that the ones with puerperal psychosis had a much shorter onset to the illness and were admitted more quickly to hospital, often within a day or two of its development, than were the control women.

In the personal survey of 413 women with postnatal depression, referred to in the previous chapter, it was noted that 51 per cent of women with puerperal psychosis had been admitted within fourteen days of the birth, while in the milder cases treated by the general practitioner the reverse was true with 39 per cent starting between the sixth week and sixth month (Figure 8).

Postnatal depression can also start after a miscarriage or termination of pregnancy, in which case it tends to occur early, within six weeks and is commonest where there has been a previous postnatal depression.

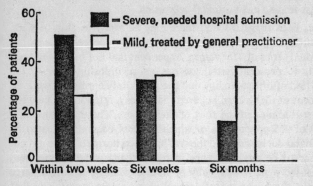

Fig. 8. Time of onset of postnatal depression in 413 patients

Effect of birth on mothers and fathers

Prof R E Kendell, now at the Royal Edinburgh Hospital, carried out a fascinating study at Camberwell, South London, to see whether childbirth had any significant effect on psychiatric illnesses of the mother and father. He scrutinized the records of all births in 1970 within the boundary of Camberwell. He then searched the parents' records for the two years before and the two years after, looking for psychiatric in-patient and out-patient consultations, and published his findings in *Mental Illness in Pregnancy and the Puerperium*. In the mother the episodes had a significant peak in the three months immediately after the birth, and a more prolonged rise later, this was particularly marked in relation to psychotic episodes compared with depressive episodes, although both were higher than expected. In contrast the fathers had a steady and low incidence of new episodes throughout the four years, and were not affected by the birth of the child.

Doctors like to talk about Couvade's syndrome, which is a psychiatric disturbance which occurs in a man during his wife's pregnancy, but Couvade's syndrome did not appear in this Camberwell study.

Breast-feeding and postnatal depression

It has been suggested that there may be a relationship between breast-feeding and the onset of postnatal depression. In my personal series of 413 women 26 per cent had not breast-fed their child, 46 per cent felt there was no relationship between the duration of breast-feeding and the postnatal depression, while 28 per cent of the women believed there was a relationship between breast-feeding and the start of their illness. These women had a total of 915 pregnancies of which 609 had been complicated by postnatal depression and the rest had been normal. There did not appear to be any difference in the outcome whether they had breast-fed a particular baby or not. Inevitably, in such a large sample, there was the occasional woman who maintained that she had been advised to stop breast-feeding and this caused her breakdown, and on the other hand a woman who felt she developed postnatal depression because she had been advised to continue breast-feeding. But on the evidence, breast-feeding did not appear to affect either the time of onset or the severity of the illness.

Pregnancy

Not all women thrive in pregnancy. A survey by the author in 1960 of over 600 women at the Obstetric Hospital, University College Hospital, London, revealed that one in four of the expectant mothers who complained of pregnancy symptoms (nausea and vomiting, depression, tiredness, backache, headache, and fainting) during the middle months of pregnancy later required admission to hospital because of high blood pressure or preeclampsia (PE). There are also a few women who find they become very depressed, sad, and hopeless during pregnancy and they may even have suicidal tendencies or develop a psychosis requiring admission to hospital. This depression, which comes out of the blue during pregnancy, may continue and develop into puerperal psychosis or postnatal depression after delivery. The doctors who are studying the hormonal changes of pregnancy and puerperium have drawn attention to the finding of depression in the last few days of pregnancy which may be heralding a postnatal depression.

Vanessa is an example of those women whose depression started during pregnancy, and it is also interesting that her mother suffered similarly. Vanessa was born in St Ebba's Hospital, Surrey, in the days when it was called a 'lunatic asylum'. Her mother had become psychotic during the pregnancy and was not discharged until six months after Vanessa was born. During both of her pregnancies Vanessa became depressed with very disturbed behaviour and had to be admitted to hospital. Vanessa's illnesses also eased spontaneously during the first year after the birth of her son and daughter.

Those who become pregnant again before their postnatal depression has eased will find that the depression lifts immediately pregnancy starts, and then it is anyone's guess whether it will return again after the next birth.

Wanda described this effect of a second pregnancy when she wrote:

'After my first child was born in 1972 I felt fine until giving up feeding her at six months. Then I became ill, imagined I was suffering from cancer or something horrific. Eventually I found myself very depressed and frightened, even of myself. On one occasion if my parents had not come round I felt I would put my head in the gas oven. A terrible feeling. I lost all my self-confidence and if we ever had to go out I would funk it and feel very sick. Eventually I became pregnant again when my child was 9 months old and then suddenly everything went. I was on top of the world once more.'

Women who suffer from premenstrual depression and tension with its wide variety of symptoms ranging from depression and tension to asthma, migraine, and epilepsy, may well find that the first sign of pregnancy is the relief of their symptoms, which usually occurs within the first month, but certainly before the fourth month is reached.

Termination of pregnancy

During the early months of an unplanned pregnancy there may be that terrible 'Shall I? Shan't I?' quandary. This is a time when there is depression mixed with anxiety, shame, and anger, and a lot of hard thinking is going on trying to decide whether she can, or should, have the pregnancy terminated or let it continue normally. If the pregnancy is terminated it may be followed by guilt, and postnatal depression can still occur, especially in a woman who has previously had a postnatal breakdown. Or there may be a short-lived period of exhaustion, partly the result of the abrupt alteration of hormone levels that the abortion brings, and also due to having insufficient rest and time to adjust afterwards. The favourite time for terminations is at the weekend so that the woman can go straight back to work without those in her office knowing of her predicament. But with the rapid resumption of work she may have a heavy price to pay.

Sometimes the request for an abortion is refused, and then the distressed mother may find a back-street abortionist who will oblige. Or the depression may get blacker and the psychiatrist may have to revise his opinion and agree to terminate. On the other hand if she changes her mind and accepts the pregnancy the depression usually lifts and may give way to a sense of elation.

Tragically, but rarely, one meets a woman who has been struggling for several years to become pregnant but when she finally succeeds, the pregnancy symptoms with daily vomiting and deep depression get too much for her and she pleads for her pregnancy to be ended. Annabelle was 31 years old when, after attending one of the Infertility Clinics at a London medical school, she asked for such help when she was ten weeks pregnant: 'I can't go on', she pleaded amid tears and sobs, 'No one knows what it's like. No one told me it would be like this. I'm ready to end it all if you don't help me.'

She needed treatment to ease her frequent vomiting and depression, and agreed to a four day trial of progesterone. This soon lifted the daily vomiting, and common sense prevailed. She later was delivered of a fine boy, whom she called after the name of the medical school which helped her to become pregnant.

Sterilization

Sometimes sterilization is blamed for the onset of a depression, but this will not cause a hormonal depression because no hormones are involved in the simple operation designed to block the

Fallopian tubes. More often, on fuller inquiry, it will be discovered that the sterilization was performed after a pregnancy and the woman is suffering from postnatal depression, or it was performed after a termination of pregnancy and it is a post-abortal depression. On the other hand the woman may have been on the Pill until the operation, and may then find on stopping the Pill that menstruation is heavier, irregular, and complicated by the premenstrual syndrome and depression.

11
The premenstrual syndrome

The next question to be answered is 'When will it ever end?' This was asked by two women because:

'After four years there is still no sign of the depression, which started so suddenly and without invitation after my baby's arrival, making a permanent exit.'

'I am now 42 years of age and have been plagued by a multitude of physical and emotional symptoms that started and became worse after the birth of my son and my daughter.'

While maternity blues and postnatal exhaustion are self-limiting, the postnatal depression and psychosis can go on for years. The psychosis is treated in hospital sufficiently to allow the woman to function in the community, and the majority are usually discharged within a few months. But too often they are far from well and still need continuous drug therapy.

There may be a lapse of up to nine months after the birth before menstruation returns naturally, and even then there is not necessarily a regular interval between menstruations. There is usually a warning with the deterioration of a mother's mental state for up to fourteen days before. Then after that first menstruation is over there may be some relief of depression and tension for a few days. Gradually the depression eases with the relief and improvement occurring during the few days after menstruation (known as the postmenstruum), but there is a rapid return of the unpleasant symptoms in the days before menstruation (known as the premenstruum). This is represented as Stage 2 on Figure 9, and the patient may remain in this stage for many years with continuous depression increasing in the premenstruum.

If improvement continues, full relief will come imperceptibly with a return of normality during the postmenstrual days; such a pattern represents the premenstrual syndrome, or Stage 3 in Figure 9. As improvement continues the episode of premenstrual depression may slowly decrease, not lasting for so long and not being quite so incapacitating, until perhaps it only lasts for one or two days before menstruation. This is the stage which was described by one husband, a building contractor, who said about his wife:

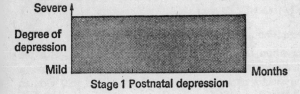

Stage 1 Postnatal depression

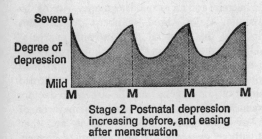

Stage 2 Postnatal depression increasing before, and easing after menstruation

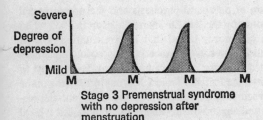

Stage 3 Premenstrual syndrome with no depression after menstruation

M = menstruation

Fig. 9. Stages as postnatal depression changes to the premenstrual syndrome

'She has a lot of up and down aspects to her character, and at the moment they really seem to have settled into monthly glooms and highs.'

However, these mood swings from improvement in the post-menstruum to deep despair in the premenstruum do not necessarily improve and they may continue for twenty or more years, until the menstruating years end with the menopause. This must be recognized as the premenstrual syndrome, which can be successfully treated.

Early recognition of the effect of menstruation

The observation that postnatal depression may start with the first menstruation after childbirth was made by Dr Marcé, a French physician, as long ago as 1855. He noted that women whose postnatal depression started with the return of their menstruation frequently complained of vagueness, poor memory, weakness, pallor, anaemia, and menstrual irregularity. Across the Atlantic in Mississippi, Major Alfred Blumberg and Dr Otto Billig reported in 1942 that hospital patients with puerperal psychosis showed these same swings in their psychotic behaviour, becoming worse after ovulation until menstruation and then improving following menstruation. These findings were confirmed by Dr Harry Schmidt of Los Angeles, and the American doctors came to the conclusion that puerperal psychosis must be of hormonal origin, or have a hormonal component, and they started treatment with progesterone, the hormone of pregnancy. But more about that in Chapter 15.

This association of puerperal psychosis and the premenstrual syndrome was noted by the late Dr Joan Malleson in 1953 when she wrote: 'It is commonly found that if menstruation returns before the psychosis is resolved, exacerbations occur repeatedly in the premenstrual phase.' This caused Dr A B Hegarty to suggest in a letter to the British Medical Journal in 1955 the name 'post-puerperal recurrent depression' for the recurrent depression, irritability, and tension during an attack of mild, but typical puerperal depression, and whose symptoms are worse in the premenstrual phase. However this title would exclude those women with premenstrual syndrome whose onset was not related to puerperal depression, so his suggestion did not win wide acclaim.

In 100 consecutive patients seen at the Premenstrual Syndrome Clinic at University College Hospital, London, there had been 59 pregnancies (including 6 miscarriages) and it was found that post-natal depression of sufficient severity to require medical or psychiatric treatment had occurred in 73 per cent. Viewed from another angle, if a patient has a postnatal depression her chances of subsequently developing the premenstrual syndrome are nearly 90 per cent.

Definition of the premenstrual syndrome

It is important to know the correct definition of the premenstrual syndrome because the phrase is often used very loosely and frequently in its wrong context. The premenstrual syndrome is defined as: 'The presence of symptoms, any symptoms, which recur regularly, always in the same phase of the menstrual cycle, usually the premenstruum and early menstruation, followed by several days entirely free from symptoms.'

Using this definition you will understand why Stage 2 on Figure 9 could never be the premenstrual syndrome because the depression continues during the postmenstruum. It is only in Stage 3, when there is no depression in the postmenstruum, that the title premenstrual syndrome can correctly be used.

The word 'syndrome' means a collection of symptoms which commonly occur together. In the premenstrual syndrome there are a great variety of symptoms which can be included, such as headaches and migraine, backache, joint pains, bloatedness, asthma, hay fever, and epilepsy. These symptoms of course occur in men and children, but they are only included in the premenstrual syndrome if there is the correct time-relationship with menstruation and if there are a few days completely without symptoms, always at the same phase of each menstrual cycle.

Tension, which includes tiredness, depression, and irritability is a very common symptom complex in the premenstrual syndrome, so much so that when only tiredness, depression, and irritability occur in relationship to menstruation it is called 'premenstrual tension'.

The more one appreciates the characteristics and common symptoms of the premenstrual syndrome the easier it is to understand the similarities between this syndrome and postnatal depression. Tiredness, depression, and irritability are all common symptoms of postnatal depression. Water retention occurs in the premenstrual syndrome which results in bloatedness and weight gain, and can be responsible for the generalized aching of bones, muscles, joints, and also for headaches. There is premenstrual retention of sodium and loss of potassium, and if the potassium is too low it causes exhaustion and weakness of the limbs. There is altered glucose tolerance during the premenstruum so that the individual becomes more sensitive to a reduced blood sugar level, and when a low level occurs it is automatically restored by the outpouring of adrenalin into the blood, which can account for sudden panics, aggressive outbursts and irritability, faintness, and migraine. Again the increased appetite and sugar cravings, the binges and food cravings can all be understood. There is a remarkable similarity of symptoms in both the premenstrual syndrome and postnatal depression, in fact many of the quotations given earlier could also apply to women suffering from the premenstrual syndrome, so long as the symptoms occur only before menstruation and completely disappear after menstruation is finished.

A fuller description of the many symptoms of the premenstrual syndrome is to be found in *Once a Month* by the same author.

Diagnosis of the premenstrual syndrome

To decide whether an individual woman suffers from the premenstrual syndrome depends not on the many and different symptoms she can recount, but on the timing of the symptoms in relationship to menstruation. Therefore it is no good going to a doctor and asking for help for the premenstrual syndrome unless you can take with you an accurate record of the times of your troubles and absence of troubles, and the dates of menstruation. Our menstrual patterns are all different. Sometimes menstruation comes every three weeks and sometimes every five weeks, in some menstruation only lasts two days and in others it lasts seven or eight days, so a menstrual record is essential. Although there are

Day	Jan.	Feb.	Mar.	Apr.	May
1			T	T	T
2			T	T	M
3			T	T	M
4			T	T	M
5			TQ	T	M
6	T		TQ	MQ	
7	T		TQ	M	
8	TQ		MT	M	
9	T	T	MT	M	
10	T	T	M		
11	T	T	M		
12	T	T			
13	T	T			
14	T	MQ			
15	TQ	M			
16	TQ	M			
17	MT	M			
18	M				
19	M				
20					
21					
22					
23					
24					
25					
26					
27				T	
28				T	
29				T	
30				T	
31					

Day	Jan.	Feb.	Mar.	Apr.	May
1					
2					
3					
4					
5					
6					
7					
8					
9					
10					
11					
12				T	
13				T	
14	T	T		T	T
15				T	
16	T		T	T	T
17	T	TH	T	T	T
18		T	T	TH	T
19	TH	TH	T	TH	MT
20	TH	M	T	TM	M
21	T	M	TH	HM	MH
22	TM	M	T	M	MH
23	M	M	MH	M	M
24	M	M	M	M	M
25	M	M	M	M	M
26	M		M		
27		M			
28		M			
29					
30					
31					

M = Menstruation T = Extra tired

Q = Quarrels H = Headache

Fig. 10. Chart for recording the premenstrual syndrome

many different kinds of charts on which such records can be kept, a useful one for this purpose is shown in Figure 10. All that is necessary is for you to mark with an 'M' the days of menstruation (or 'P' for period if that is what you call it), and then devise other symbols to denote your various symptoms, such as 'H' for headaches, 'Q' for quarrels and loss of temper, 'T' for those days when you really feel flaked out with tiredness. These charts can also be useful for postnatal depression, to record the gradual change to the premenstrual syndrome, as shown in Figure 11.

Belinda had her first baby in January. Previously she had suffered from the premenstrual syndrome, so she was used to recording the days of her tension, which before pregnancy only lasted for two days. She was entirely free from maternity blues, but then depression started in early April, rapidly becoming worse. She had her first menstruation after childbirth in May, which was preceded by an increase in depression, and she became very irritable for six days, but there was some improvement after menstruation. The progress continued and after her July menstruation she had a few days when she felt really well for the first time in three months. It wasn't long before the gloom again descended. But gradually the brighter days lasted longer and the premenstrual tension was not too bad. At last she sought treatment in November, and her problem was solved.

Women plagued with the premenstrual syndrome naturally seek a permanent solution to their monthly problems. It is all too easy to imagine that the removal of the womb, the source of the menstrual bleeding, will end their recurring miseries. After all a hysterectomy is relatively safe and frequently performed, and although it is a major operation most women leave hospital within two to three weeks. Unfortunately a hysterectomy is not the answer to the premenstrual syndrome. The menstrual hormones are controlled by the menstrual clock, situated at the base of the brain, and whether the womb is present or absent the menstrual clock and the pituitary will continue methodically to produce the stimulation that pours the menstrual hormones into the bloodstream. If there is an imbalance of menstrual hormones sufficient to cause the symptoms of the premenstrual syndrome, then even after a hysterectomy the same imbalance of menstrual

	Jan.	Feb.	Mar.	Apr.	May	Jun.	Jul.	Aug.	Sep.	Oct.	Nov.	Dec.
1					X	X M	•		•	•		
2					X	X M	•		•	•	•	
3				•	X	X	•		•	•	•	
4				•	X	•	•		•	•	X	
5				•	X	•	•		•	•	X	
6				•	X	•	•	•	•	•	X	
7				•	X	•	•	•	•	X	X	
8				X	X	•	•	•	•	X	X	M
9	Baby			X	X	•	•	•	•	X	X	M
10				X	X	•	X	•	X	X	X	M
11				X	X	•	X	X	X	X	M x	M
12				X	X	x	X	X	X	X	M x	
13				X	X	x	x	X	X	X	M	
14				X	X	x	x	X	X	M	M	
15				X	X	x	x	X	X	M		
16				X	X	x	x	X	M	M		
17				X	X	x	X	X	M x			
18				X	X	x	X	X	M x			
19				X	x	X	X	x M	M x			
20				X	x	X	X	x M	M x			
21				X	x	X	X	x M	•			
22				X	X	X	x M	x M				
23				x	X	X	x M	x M				
24				x	X	X	x M					
25				x	X	x M	x M					
26				x	X	x M	x M					
27				x	X	x M	x M					
28				x	X M	x M						
29				x	X M	x						
30				x	X M	x						
31					X M			•				

M = Menstruation   • = Mild depression

x = Moderate depression   X = Severe depression

Fig. 11. Chart showing change from postnatal depression to the premenstrual syndrome

hormones will persist and produce regular symptoms at monthly intervals without menstruation. There is a better treatment for the premenstrual syndrome than hysterectomy such as correcting the hormonal imbalance with progesterone.

Recognition of the similarities between postnatal depression and the premenstrual syndrome will open the door to more successful treatment of postnatal depression, but it requires an understanding of the hormonal changes of menstruation, pregnancy, and the puerperium, which are dealt with in Chapter 12.

12
Hormonal upheaval

Hormones are chemical messengers in the body, which produce changes in selected cells. The definition of a hormone in *The Shorter Oxford English Dictionary* states: 'Substance formed in an organ and serving to excite some vital process, as secretion'. Hormone is derived from a Greek word meaning 'to urge on', which is exactly what hormones do? they urge on certain cells to do particular tasks. Hormones are produced in one organ, called an endocrine gland, and pass in the blood to act on some other organ at a distant site. This is why those who specialize in the study of hormones are called endocrinologists. Hormones are very powerful and only minute quantities are needed to produce profound effects. They are also very selective, usually only having a few tasks to perform, and are only able to work if the conditions are exactly right.

All the body's activities are controlled by hormones. They control our growth, temperature, reactions to stress, digestion, excretion, pigmentation, and many other functions, but in this chapter we are only concerned with the hormones involved in the purely feminine functions of menstruation and pregnancy.

The pituitary gland, situated next to the hypothalamus at the base of the brain, was once called 'the leader of the endocrine orchestra' because it controlled so many hormones and was responsible for so many functions of the body. But now that we have a greater appreciation of the importance of the hypothalamus and its intimate relationship with the pituitary, we refer instead to the hypothalamic-pituitary axis and we are no longer so sure as to which organ holds the seat of greatest power (Figure 12).

The hypothalamus contains the menstrual control centre (the menstrual clock), and also the controlling centres for mood,

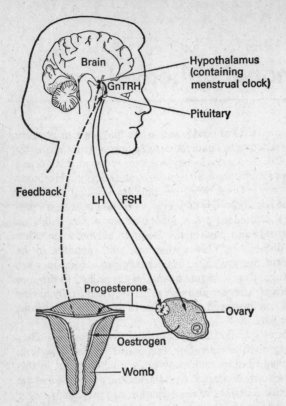

Fig. 12. Diagram of menstrual hormones showing position of hypothalamus and pituitary

sleep, weight, and day/night rhythm. Some readers will need no reminding that during postnatal depression the mood, sleep, weight, and day/night rhythm are disturbed.

In normal menstruating women the menstrual clock is responsible for releasing the necessary hormones to regulate the timing of ovulation and menstruation, and deciding the intervals between menstruations, but in pregnancy this controlling function is no longer needed as the control of pregnancy hormones is taken over by the placental-foetal axis, and the menstrual clock enters a temporary dormant phase.

The hypothalamus produces a very powerful hormone, called gonadotrophin releasing hormone, or GnRH, which passes by a special pathway to the pituitary, where it stimulates the release of two menstrual hormones called follicle stimulating hormone or FSH, and luteinizing hormone or LH. From the pituitary FSH passes in the blood to the ovary where it has two functions. It causes one of the thousands of immature follicles within the ovary to ripen and come to the surface of the ovary, where it appears as a little blister, and within it is the egg cell. It also stimulates the ovarian cells to produce the hormone oestrogen. This oestrogen passes in the blood to the womb, where it rebuilds the inner lining which disintegrated and was shed at the time of the last menstruation (Figure 12).

The other hormone from the pituitary, luteinizing hormone (LH), also passes to the ovary where it acts upon the ripening follicle causing it to burst and release the egg cell. This is known as ovulation, and normally occurs fourteen days before the onset of menstruation. The LH also causes special cells to be formed where the follicle burst, and these cells have the remarkable property of producing the hormone progesterone. Progesterone is only present in the blood after ovulation and until menstruation. It passes in the blood to the womb, where it has the task of thickening the lining, so that if conception occurs there is a comfortable soft lining inside the womb in which the fertilized egg can become embedded. Progesterone is known as the pregnancy hormone because it prepares the womb for a possible pregnancy.

The levels of the various menstrual hormones vary throughout the menstrual cycle (Figure 13). The hormone LH is present in small amounts throughout the cycle, with a high peak of ovulation. FSH is also present throughout the cycle but its level varies. These hormones do not enter the blood-stream in a continuous flow, but in spurts. For instance, it has been estimated that in the case of LH the spurts occur at about twenty minute intervals. Oestrogen is present throughout the cycle in varying amounts, having a higher level at the time of ovulation and again half-way between ovulation and menstruation. In contrast, progesterone

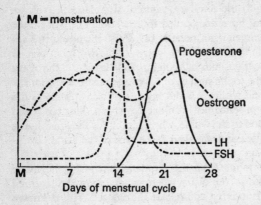

Fig. 13. Menstrual hormone variations during the menstrual cycle

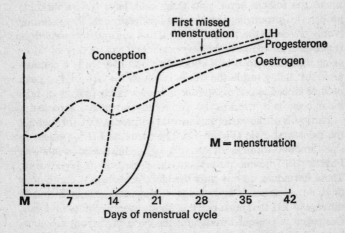

Fig. 14. Changes in hormone levels in early pregnancy

is present in unmeasurable quantities during the first half of the menstrual cycle, increasing only at ovulation. It rises to a peak half-way between ovulation and menstruation at about the twenty-first day, and then rapidly falls away, and disappears at menstruation.

Pregnancy hormones

At conception there are immediate changes in the hormone level, even before the woman has missed her first menstruation or before the foetus has become embedded within the womb. This provides justification for those women who notice the difference and are sure they are pregnant a day or two after conception and before they have missed menstruation. As one expectant mother explained:

'I knew I had conceived. First I had a terrible migraine, then within a day or two I started feeling sick and tired and my boobs became tender and bigger, but I still had to wait another seven days to see if my period would turn up. My husband didn't believe me, but I knew our baby was on the way.'

Within hours of conception the fertilized egg cell affects the hormones. The levels of LH, oestrogen, and progesterone, instead of dropping continue to rise throughout the pregnancy (Figure 14), and at least four unique new hormones are produced. They are considered unique because they have never been found except during pregnancy. They are called human chorionic gonadotrophin, human placental lactogen, human chorionic thyrotrophin, and human molar thyrotrophin. Gradually the placenta is formed and becomes a hormone factory producing massive amounts of oestrogen and progesterone during the pregnancy under the partial control of the foetal adrenal glands. During the early weeks of pregnancy this oestrogen and progesterone is produced by the ovary, but gradually the placenta takes over the production, which causes the progesterone levels in the blood to rise some fifteen to thirty times higher than the normal peak level of progesterone occurring on the twenty-first day of a non-pregnant woman (Figure 15).

Another hormone that shows a marked increase in output is prolactin produced by the pituitary. The level becomes raised

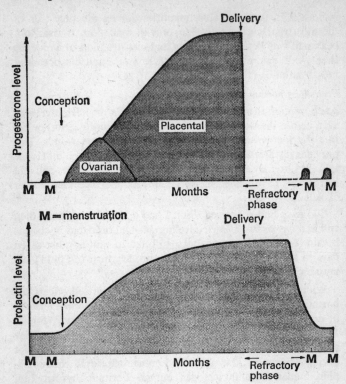

Fig. 15. Levels of progesterone and prolactin in menstruation, pregnancy, and refractory phase

throughout pregnancy and it is responsible for the preparation of the breasts for lactation. Even in the early stages of pregnancy one of the first symptoms may be an increase in the size of the breasts with the veins becoming visible, and it may be possible to express some fluid from the nipple as early as the sixth to eighth week of pregnancy.

During pregnancy the amount of hormones produced by the adrenals increases, so that twice as much corticosteroid is produced. In addition there is a change in the day/night rhythm in late pregnancy, so that more corticosteroids are produced at midnight in a pregnant woman, compared with the usual peak hour at about 9.00 am in a non-pregnant woman.

Throughout pregnancy the levels of all these hormones are controlled by the placenta and foetus, so the menstrual clock rests until menstruation restarts after the birth of the baby.

Labour

With the production of new hormones during pregnancy there is a complete change in the amounts circulating in the body, but nevertheless the changes are gradual and can hardly be compared with the sudden abrupt alterations which occur at birth when the placenta and the baby are delivered together. It has taken months to build up to these levels, but within hours the hormones drop to insignificant amounts. Only very minute quantities of progesterone and oestrogen circulate in the blood. The amounts are so small that they are measured in nanograms per millilitre, or 'ng/ml', which is 1/1,000,000,000 of a gram in a millilitre of blood. To give readers some idea of just how small that fraction is, if we equate one gram with ten million pounds sterling, then one nanogram would equal one penny. The progesterone level in the blood drops from about 150 ng/ml at the end of pregnancy to under 7 ng/ml on the third day after birth and disappears completely by the seventh day after birth. Similarly oestrogen drops from the average of 2,000 ng/ml in late pregnancy to 20 ng/ml on the third day after birth, and then levels off at about 10 ng/ml and remains at this level until the changes of menstruation occur. The four unique hormones which were produced by the placenta disappear completely. On the other hand the pituitary continues to produce large quantities of prolactin for breast-feeding (Figure 19).

A mother's normal adjustment to such marked changes in hormonal levels is indeed heroic, and one wonders at the large number of women who can stand up to the changes without upset, rather than express surprise at the few who are disturbed by this hormonal upheaval.

It is interesting that animals eat the placenta after the birth, but that cannot be to overcome the rapid drop in hormone levels as the hormones would be broken down by digestion and would be unlikely to be absorbed.

The puerperium

Once the levels of oestrogen and progesterone have dropped after delivery, the level of oestrogen remains low and there is a complete absence of progesterone. This is the resting or refractory stage during which the pituitary and ovarian response to GnRH and to LH is ineffective. Thus if the usual stimulants are given to the pituitary or ovary, such as GnRH, LH, or the fertility drug clomiphene which normally stimulates ovulation, it will not result in the normal outpouring of the appropriate hormones. The menstrual hormones of the pituitary and the ovary are resting during this refractory stage.

If the mother is breast-feeding, her prolactin level will remain raised until she stops and the refractory stage is likely to continue until then. In women who are not breast-feeding there will be a refractory stage with a raised prolactin level in the blood, which will last for about two weeks or two months, although there is considerable individual variation.

Return of menstruation

As the raised level of prolactin in the blood gradually returns to normal at the end of breast-feeding, or after a few weeks in those who have not breast-fed, there is a return of menstruation. Research workers who have done regular estimations of hormone levels from delivery of the baby onwards have been able to show that there is the expected rise of oestrogen followed by the usual peak of progesterone before the first menstruation (Figure 19). However, for some women this is when the first premenstrual tension and depression occur, while for those who have had postnatal depression this is the time of an increase in symptoms which often occur before menstruation.

There are other occasions when the menstrual clock is dormant, such as puberty, after stopping the Pill, or in anorexia nervosa, and in all these instances the premenstrual syndrome is likely to start after the dormant or refractory phase of the menstrual clock ends.

Hormonal cause

With a full appreciation of the violent upheavals which occur in a woman's hormonal system as she changes from her non-pregnant state through pregnancy, birth, puerperium, refractory stage, and back again to menstruation once more, it is no surprise to learn that for a few women it is all too much, and the result is a breakdown or postnatal depression. For some of the mothers the mental disturbances occur during the hormonal upsets of pregnancy, but for the majority it is the abrupt alterations which occur at the time of the birth that provide the trigger factor. Many women are better than usual and elated in late pregnancy, these will tend to be women with ample supplies of placental progesterone, but they will also be the ones who have the greatest difference in the levels of their progesterone in late pregnancy and early puerperium and so are most likely to develop postnatal depression.

Professor Nott and his team from Oxford University studied the hormonal levels of twenty-seven women in late pregnancy right through until after the birth. The women completed questionnaires designed to detect evidence of depression. The team found that those women with the greatest drop in progesterone levels after delivery were also those most likely to rate themselves depressed within ten days of birth, but they were less likely to report the sleep disorders so characteristic of typical depression. The pregnancy oestrogen levels tended to be higher in those women who were more irritable after delivery. Finally they found that the group of women who were depressed after the birth contained more of those who suffered from premenstrual tension. It should be noted that although depression was detected by means of a highly sensitive questionnaire, none of these were so depressed as to need medication.

Dr K McNally and his colleagues showed that prolactin inhibits the release of progesterone from those special cells where it is produced in the ovary. Drs L J Benedek-Jaszmann and M D Hearn-Sturtevant from the Regional Protestant Hospital in Bennekom, Netherlands, were the first to point out that some women with premenstrual syndrome attending the hospital's infertility clinic had raised prolactin levels. They treated the women successfully by lowering the prolactin level with bromo-criptine, and relieved their premenstrual syndrome. Madeline Munday, working at St Thomas's Hospital, London, also confirmed that in some women with premenstrual syndrome there was a high level of prolactin.

It has already been emphasized that women with postnatal depression and psychosis deteriorate during the premenstruum, which is the time when another drop in progesterone level occurs after the peak on the twenty-first day. Could it be that those women who had difficulty in coping with the abrupt drop in progesterone in early puerperium and the complete absence of progesterone during the refractory stage cannot tolerate yet another deficiency of progesterone at the time when their body needs it before menstruation?

The proverb says 'the proof of the pudding is in the eating' and progesterone has been successfully used in the treatment of postnatal depression, but more of that in Chapter 15.

The Pill

Claire, a 28-year-old hairdresser, asked:

'I would like to know why the Pill makes me feel so horrible now, yet it never caused any trouble when I used it for the four years after marriage. It's only since Ian's been born. I've tried three types and am now on ... a progestogen-only pill. But they're all the same. I feel miserable, cranky, fed up, and have become cold and frigid.'

Often after the birth women like Claire, who were able to take the Pill without trouble, later find it doesn't suit them. To understand the reason, it is necessary to know that there is a vital difference between the natural hormone progesterone and the synthetic compounds known as progestogens. They are not the same, although many people think they are. The natural hormone, progesterone, about which we've heard so much in this Chapter, cannot be absorbed when given by mouth. This also happens with some other natural hormones, for example insulin, which is used for diabetics. When progesterone is needed it is given by injection or as suppositories or pessaries. But the bio-chemists searched for something that could be given by mouth and made several completely new compounds such as one which we now know as norethisterone. When they tested it they found it was an excellent contraceptive, but it could not replace pro-gesterone in the body. It could produce vaginal bleeding when given to rats and rabbits who had their ovaries removed and had already been given oestrogen. This action is similar to progester-one and so they called it progestogen. Its formula is similar to progesterone and also similar to testosterone, the male hormone, as shown in Figure 16. Can you spot the difference? Unfortu-nately, as Dr E D B Johansson and his colleagues in Upsalla, Sweden, were the first to point out, norethisterone and the many other man-made progestogens which can be taken by mouth or used for long-acting injections all have the same action, in that they lower the woman's normal progesterone level. This means that women who are already suffering from a progesterone de-ficiency, such as those with premenstrual syndrome, are made worse when taking man-made, synthetic progestogens.

Another important difference between natural progesterone and man-made progestogens is the effect it can have on the unborn child. If the progestogens with their similarity to testo-sterone are given in early pregnancy to prevent a miscarriage they can produce an increase in male characteristics. This may not matter so much if the child is a boy, he will become more mascu-line and muscular, but if the child is a girl then the external genital organs may be changed so that at birth it is difficult to decide the sex of the baby. As the girl grows she will tend to be a tomboy. On the other hand if natural progesterone is given during pregnancy the risk of masculinization does not arise. It has been noted that mothers who are given progesterone before the six-teenth week of pregnancy have children who do well at school, especially in the science subjects. Surveys of children, whose mothers were given antenatal progesterone, have shown an educational enhancement at 9–10 years of age, at 'O' and 'A' levels, and in university entrance. One study of 34 progesterone children from the City of London Maternity Hospital showed that 32 per cent gained university admission compared with 6 per cent in control children. 6 per cent is also the average for the borough in which most of the children lived, and also for the Inner London Education Authority in which area the hospital is situated.

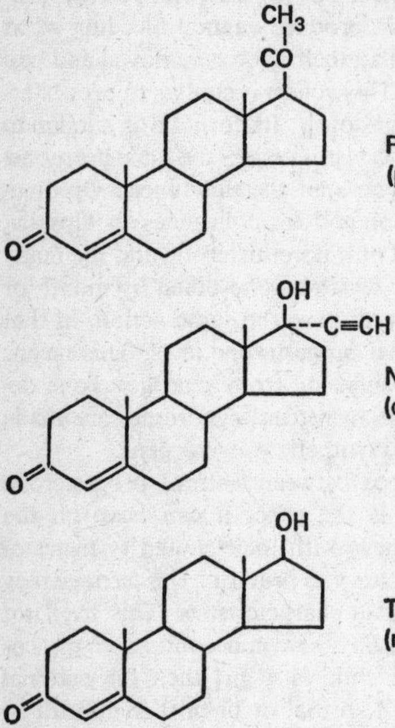

Progesterone
(pregnancy hormone)

Norethisterone
(oral contraceptive)

Testosterone
(male hormone)

Fig. 16. Which compound does norethisterone resemble?

Hormone tests

A frequent request heard by doctors is: 'Can I have my hormones tested please, so that you can find out exactly what's wrong with me?'

How one wishes the answer was as easy as that. If there is a disorder of the blood, then a blood test is invaluable. It will tell the exact number, size, and shape of your red and white blood cells. If you are anaemic a blood test will tell you exactly how much iron there is in your blood and how much iron you will need to bring your blood up to normal level. But with hormone tests it is different, particularly when dealing with tests of the menstrual hormones. Estimation of menstrual hormones are today performed by radioimmunoassay, which is an expensive and time-consuming method.

The menstrual hormones vary in amount during the menstrual cycle, thus FSH and LH peak at ovulation while progesterone peaks half-way between ovulation and the first day of menstruation, and these are the times of the cycle that the particular hormone measurement is most helpful. If the purpose is to see whether the patient has a deficiency of progesterone it is of no value to estimate the progesterone level during the first half of the menstrual cycle when it should be absent. Another difficulty is that the length of menstrual cycles vary both between individuals and in the same woman. The average length of the menstrual cycle in normal healthy women may vary between twenty-one and thirty-five days, and it is useless to assume that the patient has a cycle of twenty-eight days. Absolute precision is needed in knowing the menstrual dates. There is also the problem of other medication which the patient is receiving, thus an estimation of prolactin or progesterone cannot be performed if the patient is taking certain drugs.

When a new test of hormones is discovered there is still a considerable amount of work needed in the development stage to determine what are the normal values, whether it is affected by the time of day, activity, sleep, sex, stress, alcohol, exercise, menstrual cycle, and different types of drugs. Also it is important that other biochemists throughout the world can repeat the test and get the same results. It is only when the results in normal people have been established and confirmed on thousands of individuals worldwide that the test can be used in groups of patients suffering from different diseases. This accumulation of knowledge is time-consuming and means that it may well be five or more years before a new test becomes routine.

Among the tests which hold promise for the future are the hormone binding tests. It is now known that various hormones,

especially oestrogen, progesterone, the male hormone testosterone, and thyroid hormones can be present in the blood in
either a free state or bound to specific globulins. The hormones
bound to globulins are unable to pass through the blood-brain
barrier, so it is only the free hormone present which passes into
the cerebro-spinal fluid and bathes the brain cells. It may be that
although an individual appears to have a normal level of a certain
hormone which affects brain metabolism, too much is bound to
the globulin and too little of the hormone is actually reaching the
brain cells. At present work is proceeding on estimations of the
sex hormone binding globulin and the cortisone binding globulin, which is very encouraging and holds great promise for the
future. One hopes and expects that today's hormone tests will be
considered crude and inadequate by tomorrow's doctors.

13
All in the mind

'When endocrinology is fully understood, there will be no place for psychiatrists.' The speaker was Hans Selye, an eminent endocrinologist whose book *Stress* was the first and foremost work on the subject. In the above quotation he was reminding his audience that the science of endocrinology was gradually discovering chemicals in the human body that were producing the mental disturbances, irrational behaviour, and so on, which had hitherto been seen as psychological disturbances dealt with by a psychiatrist. This was not heralding any conflict or contest between the two disciplines but was a signpost pointing to the distant future, where the study of psychiatry will have evolved into endocrinology like a caterpillar's transformation into a beautiful butterfly. It is in this context that this book has been written, in the hope that by applying a few endocrinological findings and some clinical observation to one small but important aspect of psychiatric illness, postnatal depression, human suffering may be relieved and normal health restored.

Early this century psychiatrists realized that puerperal psychosis, as seen in the mental hospitals, could be classified as manic, schizophrenic, neurotic, or toxic confusional states, and as such were no different from other psychotic illnesses. In particular there appears to be little difference between the occasional woman who becomes confused, deluded, or hallucinatory following a major operation and the one whose mental illness follows the birth of her child. Discussion continued until, in 1943, Dr B Jacobs declared categorically in the *Journal of Mental Science* that 'a puerperal psychosis as a clinical entity does not exist'.

Whether Dr Jacobs was right or not, it is well recognized that the crisis of a baby's birth can be a traumatic experience to the body and the mind. This may be the precipitating factor which brings a latent psychological disturbance to the surface. There may be an immature personality or a long-established maladjustment which breaks down with the stress of childbirth. The symptoms may result from negative attitudes to pregnancy which have not been permitted to reveal themselves: an unconscious aversion to birth, motherhood, or children, which have been repressed and not allowed verbal expression. It may represent a rejection of the feminine role, with a dislike of housework and motherhood, and a lack of stimulating work, bringing out into the open the battle for equality of opportunity between the sexes, with the woman adopting a male hairstyle, spurning make-up, and trying to be 'one of the boys'.

The event of birth may awaken a woman's conflict with her mother resulting in her rejection of the mother role, possibly emanating from her hatred of her own mother and the realization that she is now put in the same position.

There may be a father complex, the woman having married because she required a father figure. Now she finds her husband is the father of her child and she must accept the mature role of parenthood, but this she is unable to do.

The birth also brings the loss of the thing she has nurtured so closely within her; it is taken from her to live a life apart and she feels the loneliness and the separation acutely.

It may reflect the previous poor sexual adjustment, when her sexual desires were limited and disappointing, and now the resentment towards her husband grows.

Thus the psychiatric illness could result either from the birth trauma as a source of stress, from the birth acting as a precipitating factor in a vulnerable personality, or a long-standing maladjustment or inadequate personality which comes to the surface when the woman stops work and is left with her new baby in the loneliness of her new home.

On a television programme dealing with postnatal depression, it was suggested that the ideas for a hormonal cause of postnatal illnesses represented a minority view. But, whereas it is possible that the success of a television programme may be measured in terms of the number of people who favour it, in science the concern is not with how many people support a particular view, but as to whether it reveals a new truth, a new understanding, or throws more light on the subject.

The idea that hormones can cause psychological disturbances is not new, there are many examples in medicine. The adult with too low a hormonal output from the thyroid gland may be referred to the psychiatrist because of depression, apathy, slowness of thought, inability to concentrate, and confusion. The mind is sick, but the cause is hormonal. Similarly the individual with too high a thyroid level may go to the psychiatrist with agitation, anxiety, nervousness, and restlessness and be incorrectly diagnosed as having 'anxiety neurosis', but the illness may be corrected by lowering the thyroid level. Diabetics who overdose with insulin or forget to take the correct amount of food after their injection may develop a hypoglycaemic aggressive outburst characterized by abusive behaviour and foul language before lapsing into coma; again this is easily remedied by giving glucose or adrenalin to raise the blood sugar level.

The attitude of women on first learning that their postnatal depression may be of hormonal origin varies, as is shown by the following three extracts from letters:

'My illness after baby's birth had been blamed on my early childhood and the many spankings I received then, on possible unfaithfulness of my husband (although there is no evidence that he ever was unfaithful), and my close bond with my mother. It's a great relief to know that it is caused by my hormones, even if I can't see them.'

'It is a most frustrating thing to think that perhaps my moods and desires are so controlled by my body chemistry. I like to feel I have control over myself and how I behave . . .'

'. . . and if I do find that it is not my body which does this to me, that also would be an equal relief, for at least I know what's wrong with me, I would rather be crazy and know it than live in this suicidal limbo.'

The evidence which suggests that postnatal depression is of hormonal origin relies firstly on an understanding of the tremendous hormonal changes which occur during pregnancy and the puerperium and the ease with which these various hormonal levels could be put out of balance together with an awareness of the limitation of our hormonal knowledge, which relies on measurements of hormones in the blood of the body, as opposed to the blood which crosses the blood-brain barrier and bathes the tissues of the brain, or the level of hormones within the cells of the brain. It also relies on the recognition that postnatal depression is different from typical depression, and that puerperal psychosis is different from non-puerperal psychosis. The symptomatic similarities of postnatal depression and the premenstrual syndrome coupled with the fact that postnatal depression merges into the premenstrual syndrome suggest a hormonal basis. The premenstrual syndrome is known to start at puberty, post-pill amenorrhoea, and after the amenorrhoea that occurs in anorexia nervosa, in all these conditions the menstrual clock in the hypothalamus has passed through a dormant stage.

Although there is still much more to be understood about the cause of the premenstrual syndrome, it is generally recognized to be of hormonal origin. Progesterone is effective in its treatment and is also effective in the prevention of postnatal depression and in its treatment once the refactory stage has passed and menstruation has returned.

At a conference held in London in 1978 on 'Mental Illness in Pregnancy and the Puerperium' Professor Michael Gelder, of the University Department of Oxford, said:

'It follows that while the demonstration of endocrine differences between women who are depressed and those who are not would be evidence for an endocrinal cause, failure to show a difference would not rule it out. Nor would the absence of a therapeutic response to hormones settle the point. The theory, like many others which persist in psychiatry cannot be disproved, it can only wait to be confirmed.'

14
We all can help

Deep down in everyone is a very natural desire to enjoy the best of health and generally we feel that nobody understands our problems better than ourselves. When we are unwell, as opposed to being ill, there is always a favourite personal remedy to restore us to our usual state of well-being. There is always a satisfaction in curing ourselves without the doctor's help. Some people, even when they are really ill, cling on to this desire to avoid the doctor and never is this desire greater than when there is a lurking fear that a simple visit to the health centre will result in confirmation of that unspoken fear that there really is a mental disturbance and a need to see a psychiatrist. These sentiments are expressed by Elizabeth, whose carefully penned letter says:

'As a rule I am opposed to chemicals and a believer in mind over matter. I prefer to sort myself out without assistance unless I run out of steam. Desperation causes me to seek out an alternative that might end in a solution to my problem. I have exhausted them all. Sometimes a statement only sounds so dramatic because it is true.'

That part of Elizabeth's letter might seem sensible enough but she was in desperate need of help. There is another letter, this time from a husband, who asks apologetically for help:

'I very much regret that my attitude during these scenes has obviously, with hindsight, been the wrong one and may well have exaggerated the problem, as normally I have only been able to manage frequent exhortations to "pull yourself together"; also at times of anger and violence I am ashamed to say that I, too, have been so angry myself that I have unfortunately made remarks about her mental health which naturally I now bitterly regret.

The result of such remarks seems to have been to increase the number and intensity of hysterical outbursts to such an extent that I am desperately worried as to what now we do for the best There have been occasions during the scenes when I have considered sending for an ambulance or trying to get her to the nearest hospital.'

Well, he has learned the hard and bitter way what not to do and, sadly, you cannot take back words once they have been uttered.

Heather, a 30-year-old secretary, suffered from too much advice. She meticulously listed the suggested treatments that she had been given which included: '. . . move house; – go back to work; – give up work; – you're working too hard; – take a whisky; – relax; – see a marriage counsellor; and snap out of it' when, as she said, 'all I want to do is snap out of it'.

As we have had some excellent examples of 'don'ts' in those last two letters, perhaps we should carry on with them. Here is a very basic and fundamental one:

Don't try reason on one who is mentally ill. This is a maxim that doctors and all who work with or help the mentally ill learn very early. Mental illness defies logic or reason. The mentally ill person is no longer capable of reasoning on normal thinking lines, just cast your mind back to the chapter on Nancy's Tale and remember that to Nancy's disturbed mind coincidences were everywhere, in the television programme, the apples mother brought, the porters in their black uniforms with red bands round their caps and lapels. So don't add to the complications by trying to make her see reason where, for her, reason does not exist. Postnatal depression is no different in this respect than other depressions. It is no good trying to argue that there is no need to be frightened of spiders, of going out or of staying in, of letting the baby cry or go to sleep. It is pointless assuring her that there are no dangers involved for she will still be frightened. Her thinking has become illogical, and that is that. How reason can be lost in respect of one factor but not others is seen in Jenny's story.

Jenny is the wife of a bank manager. She was frightened of travelling in any vehicle which she couldn't get out of if and when she wanted to. This precluded her from travelling by rail, 'plane, or boat, although she didn't mind going by car if her husband was driving because he would stop when asked. This limited her holidays to British resorts which could be reached by car. One day a lump was noticed in her breast. She knew and fully appreciated what breast cancer was, for her kindly mother and her much-loved step-mother had both been nursed by Jenny through the horrifying last stages of breast cancer. Realizing that she had breast cancer in no way frightened her and she accepted the diagnosis without any anxiety, but she remained frightened of travelling in enclosed vehicles.

Don't adopt a smug attitude, so giving the mother a feeling of guilt or ingratitude, rather let the mother express her true feelings of anxiety and fear.

Kay, after she had recovered, was able to recall:

'I was very irritable to my two other children and my husband. But how could I tell him how I felt? I was thoroughly ashamed and guilty of feeling like this, and he would have thought me mad, although I was not. (I have felt like it at times, though.) So I covered up except for telling my sister, who understood as she had a boyfriend who had had a breakdown and she had visited quite a few psychiatric hospitals.'

Don't nag, maybe you will need the patience of Job to repeat endlessly: 'no I don't mind that it's a boy, although before I said I wanted a daughter', – 'Baby is quite alright', – 'I really do understand that it's not your fault'. Nagging by outsiders is even worse, particularly if it comes from the older generation who have long forgotten the anguish, or from those who have never experienced it.

Don't point out her shortcomings, the unfinished jobs, or her unkempt appearance, and it doesn't help if you're forthright and say just what you think of the young mother's self-indulgence.

Don't use such glib and meaningless phrases as: 'Pull yourself together'; 'You don't know how lucky you are'; 'There are lots worse than you'; 'It's no use moaning, it won't get you anywhere'; or 'think of others'.

Don't let her be alone with the baby if you feel there is even the slightest possibility of her doing harm to it or to herself.

Don't let her feel that she is being lazy if she is resting. If she wants to go off to sleep at 7.00 pm so much the better. Sleep never did anyone any harm and she probably needs all the sleep that she can get. But if she has been given sleeping tablets, keep a careful count and hide them away. It's much too easy to swallow an extra one, and then just one or two more.

Don't say 'A new baby, my – aren't you lucky' when she feels absolutely frightful, and don't expect to see all new mothers radiating joy and contentment all day long. If you're a visitor don't stay too long – she may be longing to go to sleep again.

When coming to the list of 'Do's' mention must be made of the solution discovered by one woman who wrote: 'After my first breakdown I came to an arrangement with my husband – he agreed to give me unlimited champagne during the second week of my puerperium and all went well.'

I suppose it is better to have the head swimming from champagne than from anything else, but the mind boggles.

Do allow the new mother to talk freely and express her innermost fears without showing shock or amazement. Often there are no grounds for her fears, but let her speak about them, she needs to get them out of her system. Do show consideration and sympathy for her in her predicament.

To the mother I would say, do accept help from others, and if this is not readily forthcoming do go out of your way and enlist help. If you are lucky enough to be in the right spot at just the right time you may be able to get help from a self-help group. One such group is MAMA, the Meet-A-Mum-Association. It is a practical organization set up especially to help those mothers with baby blues. It has a nationwide network of mothers' groups which meet together over a cup of tea and chat about their anxieties, fears, loneliness, and so on with mothers who have the same fears, anxieties, and problems. There is always someone ready to chat even if it is at the end of a telephone. It is sponsored by *Woman* magazine. Other groups are run by the National Childbirth Trust, also mothers who've been through the problems of the aftermath of birth and are ready to lend a listening ear at any time of the day or night. If there aren't any members of the family or friends available to spare the odd hour it is worth contacting the local social worker or district nurse, they are usually able to find the right sort of help.

The new mother should not be ashamed to ask others to take the baby away when he's crying, it can be very disturbing to a mother who's feeling below par. It has even been suggested that there should be nurseries available for very young babies where they can be nursed by someone not emotionally involved and able to give plenty of tender loving care.

Relatives and friends need to have an infinite supply of patience and understanding, this applies especially to husbands, who may find it all beyond their comprehension and feel they cannot condone illogical behaviour.

The husband does need to wait until the depression is over and done with before beginning to make decisions. Once recovery has taken place, then is the time to decide whether to move house, change the job, build that extension to the lounge you're always talking about, and plan your holidays. It is then, in a calm and collected manner, that you can discuss plans together and make decisions that will not have to be overthrown the next day.

Do see that she avoids heavy shopping and housework. Remember those tummy muscles which were so stretched during the pregnancy – now is the time to give them a chance to recover. Certainly it's worth doing the postnatal exercises, so long as her energy permits. The worst thing is standing for too long, like standing waiting for the kettle to boil when she could be sitting down. On the other hand, if she has the energy and is houseproud, then scrubbing the floor on hands and knees is excellent for those flabby abdominal muscles.

When it comes to the matter of contraception, do consider it carefully together. If she is still depressed and has not recovered her usual *joie de vivre* then it is the husband's responsibility to ensure the necessary protection. It is not worth starting on the Pill until full recovery has occurred (see Chapter 12). This applies even if she benefitted from the hormones in the Pill before pregnancy.

Do see she has regular food, even if it's only little and often. This is not the time for dieting, the excess weight will disappear naturally without much difficulty once she feels better. At times of hormone imbalance the mother becomes especially sensitive to the blood sugar levels. Remember that the body is able to use starch as well as sugar to raise the blood sugar, so if she's not got a sweet tooth she will still benefit from savouries like potato crisps, macaroni, and crispbread. When food is eaten the blood sugar rises and then gradually drops over the next two to four hours. When the blood sugar is too low, because no food has been taken for a time, humans have an ingenious regulating mechanism which spurts adrenalin into the bloodstream and acts by releasing some of the sugar stored in the body cells to raise the blood sugar level. This spurt of adrenalin has different effects on different people, but it often causes a sudden outburst of aggression or depression, an acute panic state with a feeling of faintness, pallor, and sweating, or it may produce a migraine. The answer is simple, eat little and often, every two or three hours.

Do help the new mother to realize that, until she has fully recovered from the effects of childbirth, rigid crash dieting to restore her weight to the prepregnancy level is unnecessary. It is far better to persevere with those specially designed postnatal exercises, which strengthen the abdominal muscles and flatten the bulge.

Some women who have been on the oral contraceptive pills find they get depressed, and this depression may sometimes be relieved by taking pyridoxine, or vitamin B6. This is because pyridoxine is needed in the brain for the build-up of a special chemical called tryptophan. Similarly there are some women who have the premenstrual syndrome and benefit from the correction of any pyridoxine deficiency. Pyridoxine was once thought to be harmless, but now it is appreciated that overdosage can cause problems in some women. There have been reports of it causing harm to the nerves of the arms and legs, resulting in numbness, burning, tingling, shooting pains, also increasing depression, tiredness, headaches, irritability, and bloatedness. It is likely to be positively beneficial in about one woman in fifty. If she has given it a try for a month and feels no better there is no point in continuing; it is a sign that her depression is not due to pyridoxine deficiency.

There are other women who find that they retain a lot of water and sodium, but unknown to them they also lose their potassium. A simple blood test will show who needs to take potassium tablets, and it is not wise to take large amounts of potassium if it is not needed. Women who take water tablets to reduce the water-logging and feel very tired would be advised to ask for a blood test to find out their level of potassium. Extra potassium can be taken in the diet, especially by eating bananas, and drinking tomato- and orange-juice.

A greater recognition of the problems which may follow child-birth should be part of health education. It should be included in those antenatal classes which are attended jointly by the husband and wife, it should be thoroughly understood by all paramedical staff, and there has even been a plea for schoolchildren to be taught about it in parenthood classes.

Finally, the biggest 'do' of them all for the mother, her rela-tives, and friends. Do know when to call in a doctor and spill out your trouble to him. Don't assume that he's too busy to listen to you and please realize that there is a lot that the doctor can do which can't be achieved by others. If there have been some good days among the darkness, it is well worth while the husband diligently making a note of the good and bad days, and also any days of menstruation, if this has restarted. A well-kept record can help the doctor diagnose your problems more quickly and pre-cisely.

15
Back to health

'If I could wave my magic wand and remove only one of your many problems, which one would you choose?'

This is the question patients are often asked after they have spent some time discussing the many symptoms and changes in their health since their baby was born. The most frequent reply is: 'Give me back my old energy, so that I can cope again, be bothered to do things. So that I can stay awake. Give me the energy to laugh once more.'

Loss of energy is an essential part of postnatal depression, but the medicine she is taking may be making this tiredness worse. Doctors have two favourite types of drugs which they use in the treatment of typical depression, they are the antidepressants, and the tranquillizers or sedatives. By definition tranquillizers are aimed at bringing tranquillity, calmness, and rest. The common antidepressants called tricyclics, which include such favourites as Tofranol, Tryptozol, Surmontal, Bolvidon, Prothiaden, and about another fifty names, also produce tiredness as a side effect to their main action of removing depression, so they are usually prescribed to be taken at night in the hope that the drowsiness will have passed off by the morning. One patient entered the clinic and declared: 'I've tried yellow triangles, tiny bright blue ones, red tablets, and the traditional green and black capsules, I wonder what colour you'll give me?'

It is true that if one type of tricyclic antidepressant doesn't bring any improvement after two weeks then the doctor may increase the dose or change to another type. This is good treatment for typical depression, but as the reader will appreciate, postnatal depression should NOT be treated in the typical traditional way, nor is there any justification for increasing the tiredness which is already such a problem.

The doctor must first satisfy himself that the patient is not having a recurrence of a previous depression, nor the first attack of typical endogenous depression. Having recognized it as postnatal depression and being satisfied with his diagnosis, he can then go on to treat hormonally.

The treatment to be given will depend very much on the stage at which the patient is first seen, or whether menstruation has restarted, and whether or not she is breast-feeding (see schedule of treatment). Treatment can also be given prophylactically. The possibility of the prevention of postnatal depression is an exciting new advance, and this is a good place to start discussing treatment.

Schedule of treatment

Pregnancy	Arrange prophylactic progesterone treatment to start in labour
Early puerperium	Progesterone injections, later change to suppositories
Refractory phase	Antidepressant drugs, eg monoamine oxidase inhibitors Progesterone continuously Bromocriptine if not breast-feeding Stop pill
Menstruation returned	Progesterone midcycle to menstruation Antidepressant drugs in gradually decreasing doses

Prevention

The most satisfying and successful time to use progesterone treatment is as a preventative of a recurrence of postnatal depression or psychosis, which as already mentioned is likely to occur in two out of every three women who have previously needed medical treatment for postnatal depression, and four out of every five women who have previously succumbed to puerperal psychosis. It is also advisable to give it as a preventative to women who have a family history of postnatal depression.

It is of help to those like Louise, who wrote: 'My great problem is my husband's refusal to allow me to have another child after having had a severe breakdown and spending three months in hospital after our baby Terry was born.'

Where the aim is to prevent the occurrence of postnatal

depression, it is vitally important that the patient, obstetrician, midwife, and general practitioner are fully informed and know exactly how this is to be achieved.

Progesterone is given by daily injections from the onset of labour for the next seven days or until the mother returns home. She will then use two progesterone suppositories each day for the next month or until menstruation returns. The obstetrician is asked to give the progesterone while she is in hospital, although if the patient has a long ambulance journey to the hospital, arrangements are made for her to be given the first injection before getting into the ambulance. If she comes out of hospital before eight days, the midwife will give the necessary injections. When the course of injections is finished, the patient will continue the treatment by using progesterone suppositories, morning and night, for the next month or until the return of menstruation. The general practitioner is given full particulars of the dosage schedule and asked to give the patient, in advance, the necessary prescription for the ampules of progesterone for the injections and the necessary suppositories. The mother is also given written instructions and asked to get the necessary prescriptions and take it to the chemist, so that she has her supplies ready in advance, and all is set for the great day.

A successful multicentre trial of prophylactic progesterone has reported on 100 women who had previously suffered from postnatal depression. The recurrence rate was reduced to 10%.*

It is satisfying when, having arranged prophylactic progesterone treatment for some unseen patient in co-operation with all the doctors involved, one receives letters several months later saying: 'all went well this time' – 'I didn't have those silly excitable days' – 'The baby is now six months and very contented. I'm breast-feeding and feel first rate' – 'all so different from last time'.

Mandy, 31 years of age, suffered from premenstrual tension since her teens. She was very well during her pregnancy in 1974 and had a 'small for dates' baby weighing just over 2 kilos (4 pounds 12 ounces). This was immediately followed by puerperal psychosis, which required drug therapy for three years, after which she received progesterone treatment for her premenstrual syndrome and all drugs were gradually stopped. Her second

Practitioner, June 1985.

pregnancy in 1978 was normal and she felt well throughout. She was given prophylactic progesterone in hospital and later at home and there was no recurrence of postnatal depression. Unfortunately when the baby was three months old he died suddenly in a cot death. Mandy was, of course, emotionally upset, but she did not develop depression. She was again treated with prophylactic progesterone suppositories from midcycle and all was well.

Natural progesterone cannot be utilized if given by mouth, but it is highly effective if given by injections into the muscles of the buttock, or it can be given in wax pellets as suppositories or pessaries. The advantages of injections are that their initial action is quicker and one can be sure of good absorption, so they are used if there is any severity or urgency. Where the patient needs daily supervision, injections are given to ensure that a nurse or other responsible person sees her daily. This is important, for instance, when there is a risk of suicide, injury to the baby, or alcoholism. The suppositories are pellets of pure wax impregnated with natural progesterone and are inserted into the rectum or vagina. If used in the vagina they are called pessaries, but they are exactly the same and the woman is usually left to decide which way she likes best. When the suppositories reach body temperature the wax melts and the active progesterone passes through the mucous membrane and enters the blood stream. The wax does not go into the blood, but is rejected and comes out mixed with the faeces if used rectally, or out through the vagina, lubricating it on the way.

Some may fear that the natural hormone progesterone could possibly prove to be yet another cancer-producing agent. This is a false assumption on three counts. Firstly, because it has been used since 1934 and carefully monitored since 1948 without any serious side effect. Secondly, progesterone is used for treating some forms of cancer, and finally, because natural human material is not cancer-producing. The natural hormone, insulin, has been in use for over fifty years with no evidence of cancer production. Nor does the use of thyroid hormones produce a cancer risk. Thyroxine is given at birth to cretins, and continued throughout their entire life. Blood transfusions and the use of corneal grafts to restore eyesight are among many similar examples of normal human material which can be safely used. On the other hand the man-made steroids and other drugs such as stilboestral are not normally found in the human and the risk of cancer may result either directly or from the breakdown products formed when they are discharged from the body. The human has the necessary chemicals to convert active hormones into inactive ones for waste disposal. In the case of progesterone it is changed to pregnanediol, which passes out of the body in the urine or faeces. On the other hand the body does not have the necessary chemicals to convert the progestogens into the same inactive agents and they are not disposed of in the same way as progesterone.

Early puerperium

If the patient is distressed when seen within a day or two of the birth, progesterone can bring about a dramatic transformation, because it eases the sudden drop of placental progesterone. If she is very ill the progesterone is initially given by injections for about a week, then as improvement occurs the patient may be given suppositories instead, up to six a day can be used. This is continued for another two weeks and then gradually stopped, but the patient is always left with some suppositories so that she can use them should progesterone be required during the days before her first menstruation returns.

As long ago as 1945 Drs Otto Billig and John Bradley of North Carolina noticed how puerperal psychosis in their hospital patients increased before menstruation and so for their severely ill women they used shock treatment initially, followed by progesterone alone, with gratifying results. That was in the days before antidepressants were available.

Refractory stage

If the patient is seen during the refractory stage before menstruation has returned, progesterone may be given continually to prevent the increase in severity which occurs before menstruation, but help will still be needed for the depression. As postnatal depression is not the typical depression the response to tricyclic antidepressants is not good, but there are special antidepressants known as MAOIs which are most effective.

The monoamines are important chemicals in the brain cells which help in the normal control of mood, and it is when there are insufficient monoamines that depression occurs. Also, in the brain cells there are special chemical enzymes or catalysts, known as monoamine oxidases, whose task is to break down the monoamines. The MAOIs stop this chemical action of oxidation and allow the monoamines to remain in the brain cells, so lightening the depressed mood.

MAOIs are especially useful in treating atypical depressions. A great advantage is that they do not cause drowsiness, indeed they may cause wakefulness at night, so patients are advised to take their tablets early in the day. Also they do not take so long to lift the depression; whereas tricyclic antidepressants take two weeks before they are effective, MAOIs are usually effective within four to six days. However, care must be taken with their use, they cannot be used with certain tricyclic antidepressants and never with amphetamine or morphia, which means that patients who are already on tricyclics when first seen may need to be weaned off them for ten to fourteen days before treatment with MAOIs can be started. While the patient is taking MAOIs there are certain foods which are forbidden, the most important of which are cheese, Bovril, Marmite, and broad beans. Alcohol is allowed but only in very moderate amounts. This means that MAOIs can only be given to those patients who can be relied upon to abide by the list of forbidden foods and strictly avoid them. They are always given a list of forbidden foods which they collect with their first prescription. If they transgress and take even a smaller than average portion of a forbidden food they are likely to be punished with a severe headache due to a sudden rise in blood pressure. In the early days of using MAOIs, before the food restrictions were understood, there were isolated cases of brain haemorrhage after a good pub lunch of alcohol and a quarter of a kilo (8 ounces) of cheese.

Nicola was a 28-year-old lecturer who had a clean bill of health, enjoyed a healthy pregnancy, and had an easy delivery of a 3-kilo (7-pound) son. She did not breast-feed as she hoped to resume work shortly. She told me that she started crying on the third day after the birth and hadn't stopped since, four weeks later. She was in tears in my consulting room as she explained: 'How could I possibly stand up before an audience of students like this?' She was immediately started on daily progesterone injections and on MAOIs to be taken twice daily in the mornings for three days, then increased to three daily. When seen the following week she had improved, having had fewer crying bouts. Two weeks after starting treatment, menstruation returned and she felt her 'old self again'. The MAOIs were continued for a month and then reduced. Progesterone suppositories were used from midcycle till menstruation for the next two months. She was discharged after an interval of four months, taking no medication, but keeping a careful menstrual record so that if the premenstrual syndrome occurs she will be able to have treatment immediately.

During the refractory stage, if the mother is not breast-feeding she can be given the drug bromocriptine. However, bromocriptine stops lactation, so if she is breast-feeding the mother is advised to stop gradually over the next two weeks in order that she may be given it. Bromocriptine is an ergot derivative, which lowers the level of prolactin, so it shortens the refractory stage, hastens the return of ovulation and menstruation with the return of normal levels of progesterone, and increases the normal sex drive. Bromocriptine is usually prescribed as one or two tablets to be taken with food just before going off to sleep. If they are taken in the daytime, or on an empty stomach, they can cause unpleasant nausea and dizziness.

After menstruation returns

If the patient is first seen after menstruation has recommenced then progesterone is given from the fourteenth day of her menstrual cycle and continued until the beginning of the next menstruation. If the patient has a record of accurate menstrual dates and the timing of symptoms then progesterone can be individually tailored to suit her cycle precisely. All patients receiving progesterone are encouraged to keep an accurate record of symptoms and menstruation. Unless symptoms are very severe the progesterone suppositories are used, starting with one or two daily and increasing to four if necessary.

In those whose menstruation has returned but the depression

is still present continuously, with increases in severity before menstruation (Stage 2 Figure 12), the treatment is with both MAOIs and progesterone until the depression has lifted in the postmenstruum and she reaches Stage 3 or the premenstrual syndrome. Then the MAOIs will be gradually reduced and ultimately stopped, while continuing with the progesterone from ovulation to menstruation.

Pauline, a 39-year-old housewife, had Stage 2 postnatal depression, which had been lingering on for four years. On her second visit she remarked: 'One or two days I've had a glimpse of what I was like before Stephen was born. I feel like dancing in the rain.'

Other comments heard after there has been full relief of symptoms following treatment include: 'I've a return of my old courage, now I can answer back, I can look people straight in the face and insist I get the right change', and from a Canadian patient:

'I feel so peppy that I am walking places instead of taking the subway. My mind is so clear I find myself comparing prices when I shop, instead of grabbing the nearest thing so that I can drag myself home and collapse on the bed. I am now full of ideas, and I can even discipline myself to get dreary jobs done instead of making excuses. I know I must look well because everyone is asking where I have my hair done.'

'I'm as right as rain now, and now I know for sure that I'm not a neurotic female.'

Once the postnatal depression has passed into the premenstrual syndrome the treatment becomes that of the premenstrual syndrome, which is covered in my book *Once a Month*. For members of the medical profession the full dosages and particulars of treatment are included in my book *Premenstrual Syndrome and Progesterone Therapy*.

Stop the Pill

Apart from treatment with progesterone, MAOIs, and bromocriptine there are other considerations in treating patients with postnatal depression. They will probably be advised to stop the Pill and use some other method of contraceptive. The effect of the progestogen present in the oestrogen-progestogen pill and in the progestogen-only pill is to lower the level of natural progesterone in the blood, as discussed on page 99 and this is the reverse of what is needed in postnatal depression. Also the Pill tends to prolong the refractory stage before menstruation starts, in spite of the usual scanty withdrawal bleeding at the end of each course. It may cause post-pill amenorrhoea, encouraging the menstrual clock to stay asleep instead of working again now that pregnancy is over. Oestrogens and progestogens are known to pass to the baby in the mother's breast milk and the effect of these small doses on the baby's later life is still not known. The depression may, in fact, be caused as a side-effect of the Pill, rather than being a true postnatal depression. Women who have been on the Pill and are depressed, are advised both to stop the Pill and might try a short course of pyridoxine, but see the discussion on page 112.

Blood tests

At the patient's first visit the doctor may arrange a blood test to measure the level of progesterone, prolactin, and potassium if this is possible. The prolactin blood test cannot be taken while the patient is still breast-feeding, or if she is taking the Pill, tranquillizers, antidepressants, or sleeping-tablets. It is useful to measure the level of progesterone if the mother has not menstruated since childbirth, as it gives an indication whether menstruation is to be expected during the next two weeks. If menstruation is due it could account for any increase in symptoms which may be present at that time and such symptoms should not be blamed on to any treatment she has received. If menstruation has already started a progesterone test is of no value during the first two weeks after the beginning of menstruation when progesterone is absent. Progesterone estimations are best performed seven days after ovulation, if exact menstrual dates are known. Potassium estimation is necessary if the woman is receiving a diuretic to make her pass more urine; if she is very waterlogged or has excessive exhaustion. A low potassium level may account for undue tiredness and weakness of the legs. It is possible that the doctor will also arrange blood tests to exclude any symptoms due to anaemia, thyroid deficiency, or any other disorders he may suspect.

Puerperal psychosis

In cases of severe psychosis the mother needs admission to hospital, and the sooner the better. The patient will initially need sedation to ease her confused mind and usually one of the major tranquillizers, such as Stelazine or Largactil, are given. These are valuable for the treatment of disturbed behaviour, but occasionally they cause a slight tremor or rigidity of movements, in which case other special tablets are given to remove or prevent these side effects.

Sometimes the patient has manic depression, that is when there are violent mood swings, from being unduly high with restless agitation, non-stop talking and wild flights of fancy, to a deep depression. Such psychotic patients may benefit from treatment with lithium, which is a mineral that is normally present in our blood, but only in minute traces. Lithium is given as tablets, one to four daily, but the amount individuals absorb into the blood when a tablet is swallowed varies from one individual to another, so patients need to have frequent blood tests to find out just how much lithium is reaching the blood, and to make sure the level is not too high. The early signs of overdosage are nausea and diarrhoea and the patient is advised that should these symptoms occur the lithium should be stopped completely for one day, and then restarted at a lower dose.

Long-term drug therapy

Patients with psychosis are usually not completely recovered when they are discharged from hospital. They are greatly improved, but still taking drugs, so they need careful supervision with a gradual reduction of drugs over the next few months. However, it is not unusual to meet women who have stopped seeing the psychiatrist at his hospital out-patient clinic and just continue asking the family doctor for repeat prescriptions. The family doctor is often under the impression that the patient is still seeing the psychiatrist. Some women continue for years on the same dose, and are fearful of any reduction or alteration after having taken them for perhaps ten years. Women taking antidepressant drugs do need to be supervised at intervals, so that their progress can be monitored with the aim of gradually reducing, and ultimately stopping, treatment. When reducing drugs, careful timing is needed to lower the dose immediately after menstruation when the patient is feeling her best. Often the daily dose of drugs is being continued because of the premenstrual syndrome for which the women should be using progesterone alone during the second half of their menstrual cycle.

Drugs and breast-feeding

When treating a mother who is still breast-feeding, consideration needs to be given to the effect of those drugs which are known to pass through the mother's breast milk. The most likely ones are valium, tricyclic antidepressants, oestrogens and progestogens as in the Pill, diuretics, and lithium. If valium is given the baby's progress needs careful monitoring to ensure he does not become too sleepy. If lithium is given the baby's blood also needs measuring for the level of lithium.

Future hopes

Experimental work is going on trying to find out how effective it will be to give progesterone by nasal spray. Already we know that this is a useful way of administration in monkeys and it is now being tried out on women. It is being used, under the auspices of the World Health Organization, in a trial at the Department of Anatomy at Birmingham University, and also by scientific groups in America and India. In the first place the trial is of the small dose needed to suppress ovulation, to determine if it has any use as a contraceptive when taken before ovulation. The work is being followed with interest by many women with the premenstrual syndrome, who have benefited from progesterone injections or suppositories.

Further advances in the treatment of postnatal depression depend on the biochemists devising reliable tests for the diagnosis and differentiation of the different types of depression and for monitoring the patient's progress, and searching for drugs to shorten the refractory stage by stimulating the dormant menstrual clock.

16
A way ahead

Babies should bring happiness but if they do not something is wrong. This book is an attempt to help when things do go wrong.

In the fourth century BC Hippocrates described the illness in his *Third Book of Epidemics* in which there is a reference to a woman who became restless and could not sleep, and became delirious eleven days after giving birth. She became comatose and finally died on the seventeenth day. Hippocrates suggested two causes for her illness. The blood discharges from her womb could have been carried towards her head, resulting in agitation, delirium, and attacks of mania, or 'when blood collects in the breast of a woman, it indicates madness'. These hypotheses were accepted as dogma for the next 2,000 years.

The madness aspect placed it in the realm of the psychiatrists, who treated the illness on the traditional lines of typical depressive illnesses or psychoses. We are at last emerging from that era into a new one arising out of the development of endocrinology, which is trying to understand the influence of the hormones, their interactions, and the way they affect our lives. We live in a scientific age with computerized diagnosis and sophisticated biochemical technology, but the age of clinical observation is not yet past. It was clinical observation that spotlighted the foetal damage resulting from rubella and the administration of thalidomide in early pregnancy. Again, it is clinical observation that has brought a new understanding and treatment for postnatal depression.

Observation in surgeries, health centres, and clinics will reveal the high incidence of postnatal depression and the resultant unhappiness and disruption of marriages, families, and homes. Clinical observation has formed the basis of this book and linked it with an appreciation of the hormonal upheaval in pregnancy and the puerperium which, in some women, causes this misery of miseries out of which arises the premenstrual syndrome. Paradoxically it was work on the premenstrual syndrome that brought the recognition of the similarity of postnatal depression and the relationships between the two. The successful treatment of the former with progesterone has led to the prevention and treatment of the latter. This should be a step forward in lowering the incidence of postnatal illness.

Drs Clarke and Williams, writing in the *Lancet* in 1979, estimated that each year 23,000 women in England and Wales suffer from moderate or incapacitating postnatal depression, bringing unhappiness and distress to new mothers. Surely the time has come for an increased awareness of all that is contained in this book and a concerted attempt made to erradicate the problem by a greater emphasis at the antenatal clinics on any previous psychiatric illness in the patient or the female members of her family, and a continuous observation of the psychological well-being of the woman during her pregnancy. This would enable potential sufferers to receive treatment at the earliest possible stage. There is also a need for the institution of a three- or six-month postnatal examination designed to detect, diagnose, and help the unfortunate mothers. It is hoped that from this small acorn of observation a mighty oak tree of knowledge will grow.

In tribute to the many women, whose sufferings have contributed so much to this book two of their quotations will provide the ending:

'I feel at last I can see a light at the end of a very long road.'
'I've come out of the end of the tunnel – what a wonderful surprise.'

Further reading

Dalton, K, *Premenstrual Syndrome and Progesterone Therapy* (William Heinemann Medical Books, 2nd edition 1984).
—— *Once a Month* (Fontana Paperbacks and Harvester Press, 1978).
'Prophylactic progesterone successfully used in Postnatal Depression' *Practitioner*, June 1985
Sandler, M (ed), *Mental Illness in Pregnancy and the Puerperium* (Oxford University Press, 1978).

Glossary

Abortion: death of foetus.

Adrenal glands: two glands above the kidney responsible for producing numerous hormones.

Adrenalin: one of the hormones produced by the adrenal glands.

Amenorrhoea: absence of menstruation.

Anorexia: loss of appetite.

Antenatal: before childbirth.

Antidepressant: drug to remove depression.

Anus: exit from the alimentary tract, or back passage.

Atypical: not typical.

Bromocriptine: drug which lowers prolactin level.

Cervical smear: test for the diagnosis of cancer of the neck or door of the womb.

Cervix: door of the womb.

Contraception: prevention of pregnancy.

Corticosteroids: hormones produced by the cortex of the adrenal glands.

Diuretics: drugs capable of increasing the amount of urine passed.

Dormant: sleeping or inactive.

Dyspareunia: pain on intercourse.

ECT: electroconvulsive therapy; a type of therapy in which an electric shock is administered to the brain.

Endocrine gland: organ releasing hormones into the blood to act on distant cells.

Endocrinologist: a person who studies the hormones of the body.

Endogenous: arising from within.

Endometrium: inner lining of the womb.

Exogenous: arising from outside.

Follicle stimulating hormone: hormone produced by the pituitary acting on the ovary to ripen the follicles and produce oestrogen.

Galactorrhoea: fluid in the breast when not breast-feeding.

Glucose: a form of sugar found in the blood.

Gonadotrophin: hormone produced by the pituitary acting on the gonads, either testes or ovaries.

Gynaecology: study of diseases of women.

Haemorrhage: loss of blood, bleeding.

Hormones: chemical messengers, produced by glands and having an action on cells in another part of the body.

Hypothalamus: specialized part of the base of the brain.

Infanticide: killing of an infant by its mother.

Labour: birth of baby.

Lactation: breast-feeding.

Lethargy: excessive tiredness.

Libido: sex drive.

Lithium: mineral present in the body only in minute traces.

Luteinizing hormone: hormone produced by the pituitary which causes ovulation and the production of progesterone.

Manic: mental illness with unnatural elation or excessive activity.

Maternity: related to pregnancy.

Menstrual clock: specialized portion of the hypothalamus responsible for the cyclical timing of menstruation.

Menstrual cycle: time from the first day of menstruation to the first day of the next menstruation.

Menstruation: monthly bleeding from the vagina in women of childbearing age, caused by the disintegration of the lining of the womb.

Metabolism: building up and breaking down of chemicals in the body.

Migraine: severe form of headache.

Obstetrician: specialist in the care of women during pregnancy and labour.

Oestrogen: hormone released by the ovary.

Ovary: reproductive organ containing egg cells.

Ovulation: release of egg cell from the ovary.

Ovum: egg cell.

Paramenstruum: the days immediately before and during menstruation.

Parturition: birth of the baby.

Pituitary: gland situated immediately below the brain producing numerous different hormones.

Placenta: sometimes called the 'afterbirth' – organ which develops within the womb responsible for feeding the foetus and for the production of hormones of pregnancy.

Postmenstruum: the days immediately after menstruation.

Postnatal: after childbirth.

Potassium: mineral present in blood and cells of the body.

Pre-eclampsia: illness in late pregnancy in which there is a raised blood pressure, swelling, and albumin in the urine.

Premenstruum: the days immediately before menstruation.

Progesterone: hormone produced by the ovary for the preparation of the lining of the womb, also the starting point for the production of numerous corticosteroids.

Progestogen: man-made steroid capable of causing bleeding from the lining of the womb, and having different actions to that of natural progesterone.

Prolactin: hormone produced by the pituitary gland, the most important action being concerned with breast-feeding.

Prophylactic: preventative.

Psychosis: mental illness.
Puerperium: days after childbirth.
Pyrexia: fever, raised temperature.
Pyridoxine: vitamin B6.
Refractory: resting, not easily stimulated.
Sedative: drug to bring calmness.
Sodium: mineral present in the cells and blood of the body.
Syndrome: collection of symptoms which commonly occur together.
Testes: two male reproductive organs which produce sperm and testosterone.
Testosterone: male hormone produced by the testes.
Therapy: treatment.
Thyroid: gland in the neck producing hormones responsible for the speed of metabolism of the body.
Thyroxine: hormone produced by the thyroid gland.
Tranquillizer: drug to bring tranquillity.
Trauma: injury to body or mind.
Uterus: womb.
Vagina: passage leading from the exterior of the body to the door of the womb.

Index